TESTIMONIALS

"The author succeeds in providing factual, nonjudgmental information broken down into manageable concepts. Overall the author's voice remains calm and informative, and the content doesn't appear to be sensationalistic or based on "cherry picked" data. The book should serve as a useful resource for readers interested in the topic."

– BlueInk Review

"*The 21 Unspoken Truths about Marijuana*, by Dr Antoine Kanamugire, is a timely book that falls perfectly within the present social context. What a beautiful, relevant, elegant work with the right tone. To leave in the waiting room … or in the room of your teenager!"

– Dr Evelyne Thuot, Medical Doctor, psychiatrist

"A must read for anyone that smokes cannabis or is considering using it on a regular basis. The illustrations alone included by the author tell their own story and allow you the reader to take the journey to freedom."

Fran Lewis, a Book Pleasures' reviewer and a veteran of NYC public schools, member of Who's Who of America's Teachers and Who's Who of America's Executives from Cambridge

"Thanks to the author for this great book that is easy to read and full of information relevant for everyone, especially young people aged 21 and under. All high schools should have many copies and make it a mandatory reading. Thank you also for the respectful and non-judgemental tone and the quotations filled with hope."

– Clodine Desrochers, award winning TV host, author, speaker and a mother of a teenager

"*The 21 Unspoken Truths About Marijuana* is a reference for all, it's a book that's complete and easy to understand – it really touches on many topics and spheres of life that are affected by marijuana use. The author informs with great respect for the reader and encourages a thoughtful process in order to make well-informed decisions."

– **Mélanie Canuel,** clinical nurse in psychiatry

"The *21 Unspoken Truths About Marijuana* should be distributed in schools! It could be an excellent student / teacher working tool ... It would facilitate the debate around a theme of which we have decidedly not yet finished hearing about!"

– **Mitsou Magazine (by Alexandra Filliez)**

"Easy read and very informative! The 21 Unspoken Truths about Marijuana offers critical and timely information for the public with a particular emphasis for young people. The book is also for everyone whether a user, friend, parent, brother, sister, uncle, policy maker or anyone who wants to understand the psychological effects of Marijuana. The most striking idea I retained is that if one is below 25, smoking pot might not be the best idea. The book gives information without judging anyone. I highly recommend it!"

– **Moses Garishabake,** lawyer, Board Member, Canadian Race Relations Foundation (CRRF)

"Once I started reading this book I couldn't put it down. Every home should have one or two. Easy to read and very informative. I bought three of them for my friends, just put in your home you never know it may save your kids."

– **Frédéric Ntawiniga,** Master of engineering, Senior Programmer Analyst, Federal Government of Canada

PROTECT OUR YOUTH

THE 21 UNSPOKEN TRUTHS ABOUT MARIJUANA

ANTOINE KANAMUGIRE, MD

Contents

Heartfelt Acknowledgements

First and foremost, I'd like to extend my gratitude to my precious wife Ange and our four young children, for your love, your affection, your kindness, and your unreserved support in life and throughout the process of writing this book.

On a personal note, I extend my gratitude to my older brothers for being there for me as I was growing up without a father whom I lost at a young age. Thank you for your brotherly love and untiring strength.

I am grateful for the sweet and beautiful memories of my late father, mother and sisters, who all passed so early but left me with inspiring memories filled with love, grace, courage, hope and honor.

I extend my gratitude:

To Brother Rene D. Roy, a man who tirelessly and passionately kept opening doors of opportunity for a better education, not only for me but also for several dozen young people in need. I can never express the depth of my appreciation for your love, kindness, humility, and your unwavering support throughout these many years.

To Dr. Paul Grand'Maison of the University of Sherbrooke for inspiring a whole generation of medical students through your love, affection, and through your warm presence which taught me more than words could ever hope to do. Thank you for your care and your support.

To Dr. Beatrice Granger, Dr. Guy Leveillé, Dr. Stéphane Proulx, Dr. Daniel St-Laurent, Dr. Didier Jutras-Aswad, Dr. Florence Chanut, Dr. Cedric Andrès, Dr. Michel Paradis, Dr. Francine Morin, Dr. Christiane Bertelli, Dr. Amal Abdel Baki, Dr. Rémi Coté, Dr. Mimi Israel, Dr. Serge Beaulieu, Dr. Karine Goulet, Dr. Pierre-Paul Yale, Dr. Jacques Bernier, Dr. Mylène Valiquette-Lavigne, Dr. Chantal Lemire, Dr. Don Fujito, Dr. Chris Abbott, Dr. Linda Jordan Platt and so many other mentors for your excellence in knowledge transmission, for your attention, for your support and for helping me shape my professional life.

To my former and present colleagues and collaborators from near and far, thank you for your presence, your fruitful discussions, and for your determination to make our world a better place.

I would like to thank my patients for helping me to grow not only professionally but also in my personal life. Your courage, your humility to ask for help, your perseverance and your determination to fight continues to inspire me every single day of my life.

To those of you who might be fighting the addiction of some kind, I commend your courage and personal conviction to fight for a better life.

I would like to acknowledge the efforts of those in the caring professions working tirelessly to help your patients rise above the burden of addiction. Whether you are a therapist, a doctor, a nurse, a rehab therapist, a family member, a spiritual or religious leader, or a community leader, I commend your courage and your tenacious spirit to help

Thank you to all of my friends, nieces, nephews and relatives, who help me stay balanced within this fast-paced and busy world; through your kindness, your love, your sense of humor, and the times we spend together, my life is richer and full of meaning.

I extend my gratitude to my chosen family members Denis Auray and Fleurette Morin who played a great and love-filled parental role when I needed them most.

Finally, I'd like to extend my heartfelt gratitude to Thomas Layton-Smythe, Isabelle Carrière, Viviane Cholette, Jocelyne Bouchard, Eric Moses Gashirabake, Frédéric Ntawiniga for your professionalism and contributions throughout the process of editing, creating illustrations and for your resolved support in so many other ways throughout the process of publishing and sharing this book.

Introduction

"It's easy to stand with the crowd,
it takes courage to stand alone."

—Mahatma Gandhi

I am writing this book out of love, out of passion, out of care for my fellow human beings, and out of personal duty. I feel the need to share and to engage my generation and the generations to come; I am writing to you because I believe in you! I believe in your ability to think and to cross-examine objective facts and most of all, I believe in your freedom and your capacity to learn and to make your own decisions based on your own process of investigating truth.

The idea to write this book birthed from the desire, the passion and personal mission to help inform the public about cannabis usage, and to bring about a much needed discussion about this drug with my fellow citizens of the world. As you have probably heard, several states in the United States of America have recently moved to legalize recreational marijuana usage, and Canada has legalized the sale of recreational marijuana nation-wide.

As I write, I can't help but imagine the fourteen, sixteen, or twenty-one- year-old young man or woman who might be wrestling with whether or not to try cannabis, but feel they don't have enough information to make an informed decision on one side of the argument or the other. I can't help but also consider the parents of this young person who might be wondering how to speak to their teenager about cannabis usage, or who may be struggling with whether or not to try the substance themselves.

Some people might argue that cannabis or marijuana is harmless and the proof is that it's being more and more legalized in different parts of the world, and others will argue that it's not because cannabis is being legalized that it's good for you, and they will say that tobacco smoking is legal but it remains very dangerous to your health.

This is not a book concerned with making judgements, it's not a book about telling you what to do or not to do, and it's not a book which wants to determine your choices for you; it's an informational tool using simple information and common language that anyone can understand. The intent of this book is to offer simple answers to commonly asked questions about cannabis…

What is cannabis? What changes can it make to your brain? Can it lead to mental health problems such as psychosis, depression, anxiety, or suicide? Can it lead to lung cancer? How might it affect your physical health? And what consequences might it have on your personal goals and ambitions, on your social relationships, and on your overall well-being? The goal of this book is not to judge anyone, but to provide you with illustrations, tables, basic scientific information, and easy to understand statistical tables about marijuana usage.

The purpose is to create awareness about this trivialized and supposedly harmless drug so that whatever choice we make at least we know we're making a well-advised and a well-educated choice to protect our brain, our young people's brains and to lovingly help free those who might already be oppressed by the burden of addiction.

We will mainly use the term *"cannabis"* in this book but we need to mention that *"marijuana"* is the term most commonly used around the world.

I will leave it up to you, the reader, to do the exercise of finding the *21 Unspoken Truths about Marijuana* as you progress through the reading. You may want to team up with a few other readers either directly or through a social media reading group to discuss your findings with them.

*There is a table found somewhere in the book that will help you examine whether you have explored all The 21 Unspoken Truths about Marijuana discussed in this book. That table contains all those twenty-one points.

Thank you for taking a few hours out of your precious time and hectic schedule to read and discuss the subject matter explored throughout this book, and I hope you are moved to share it with someone you care about!

Sincerely,

1

What is Cannabis?

"Drugs were a way of running from whatever it
was I wanted to run from."

**—Michael Phelps,
winner of 28 Olympic medals.**

Cannabis or Marijuana is the most commonly used addictive substance after alcohol and tobacco. It is a natural plant which causes psychotropic effects on the brain when smoked or consumed and can cause real consequences in our everyday lives. Cannabis use is a topic worth discussing since it affects so many people and is present in so many homes. It affects not only individuals, but families, communities, as well as society as a whole. Multiple social, medical, political, and legislative issues are informed by cannabis usage; recreational marijuana, medical marijuana, treatment of addiction, and legislative factors are only a few of the societal issues that need to be considered by society at large. But let's not forget that cannabis use also affects individual lives as well; cannabis can be present in your life as a simple recreational or social issue, but it can also be an addiction issue, a financial issue, a family issue as it affects your relationships with family members, or a security issue as it affects your driving capabilities.

In this chapter, we will offer some simple information about this drug, we will discuss its history, slang terms, chemical components generally found in cannabis and basic statistics about the use of marijuana in the US, Canada, and throughout the world.

Stats Corner

- Cannabis, also known as marijuana, is the most commonly used addictive substance in the world after alcohol and tobacco [2-3-4]

- Most commonly used recreational drug in adolescents and young adults in the world [3-4]

- Within the US, 22.2 million people report that they have used cannabis within the past month according to the 2015 National Survey on Drug Use and Health

- In months following cannabis legalization in Canada, there was a sharp increase in children with cannabis intoxication in a Montreal hospital.[62]

- Within Canada: usage is two to three times more frequent in youth (15-24) than in adults [5]

- Increases in teenagers' emergency department visits related to cannabis have been observed in US states that have legalized recreational marijuana [6-7]

- Increases in marijuana use by teenagers and young adults have been observed in US states that have legalized recreational marijuana [6-7]

<u>Cannabis- What is it?</u>

Cannabis, also known as marijuana, is a flowering plant. Cannabis has been used as a drug for thousands of years.

Its use has been documented dating back to more than 2500 BC by

Chinese emperors, Ancient Greeks and Romans

It's been used for recreational purposes, for medical purposes, and even for spiritual rituals in some societies.

There are three main species of cannabis: sativa, indica, and ruderalis, and these species are biologically very similar.

Sativa is the most commonly grown for recreational purposes.

While these three species might differ in heights, appearances and regions where they are more likely to grow, we will focus on their differences in terms of the effects that they produce because of their different concentrations in THC and CBD.

Sativa, has high concentration of THC, the psychoactive or mind altering chemical in cannabis that produces the 'high'. This is the most commonly grown type of cannabis and the most wanted by recreational users. Sativa has little concentration of CBD.

Indica: is more likely to have higher concentrations of CBD, hence more interesting for people looking for cannabis for medical purposes.

Ruderalis: is mostly used to produce fibers for clothing industry and seeds for animal and bird feed; some variety might contain low concentrations of CBD. It is mostly used by breeders to create marijuana hybrids that can grow in atypical environments.

Hemp: is a plant that is in the large family of cannabaceae, contrary to cannabis it contains almost no THC. It is mainly used for industrial purposes such as clothing, food, paper industries and so forth.

Slang Terms for Cannabis

Marijuana, pot, cannabis, weed, wax, stone, hash, joint, herb, mj, reefer, dope, dob

There are more than 1,000 slang names [8]

How is Cannabis Consumed?

Can be smoked like a cigarette, called a marijuana joint

Can be rolled into a cigar, called a blunt

Can be smoked through a wide glass pipe, called a bong

Can be inhaled directly, through heating marijuana or hashish and inhaling the smoke

Can be ingested directly in marijuana teas, foods, candies, cookies, or other baked goods.

Cannabis: what gets you high?

Cannabis contains more than 500 different chemical compounds. Among these chemical components are compounds called cannabinoids. These cannabinoids bind to specific receptors in your brain called cannabinoid-receptors, and there are about one-hundred cannabinoids found in cannabis.

The two main cannabinoids include: THC and Cannabidiol (CBD)

THC (tetrahydrocannabinol): This is the chemical compound responsible for getting you 'high' as well as causing other psychotropic effects.

Different THC concentrations of cannabis exist on the market.

Main cannabinoids found in cannabis

THC	CBD
Psychoactive	Not psychoactive
Mental health risks	No known mental health risks
analgesic	antiepileptic
antiemetic	Anti-inflammatory
Appetite stimulating	Neuroprotective
	Antipsychotic

And any cannabis with THC concentration above **10%** is considered **high** and potentially more harmful than cannabis with lower THC concentration.

A few decades ago Cannabis Potency or THC concentrations were much lower than they are today.

So if you feel that you absolutely have to use cannabis, at least check the concentrations of THC.

The more THC concentration in your cannabis, the more harmful to your mental health it might be.

Cannabidiol (CBD): This chemical has been mostly used for potential medical purposes.

CBD (cannabidiol), does not get you high, it is not used for recreational purposes, and it is not addictive.

CBD is being mostly used or investigated for medical usages;

CBD products may also contain some THC, so an extra level of caution is advised when taking these products.

Additionally, laboratories charged with extracting CBD from cannabis vary in their levels of accuracy.

Remember, it is not recommended to consume any drugs for medical purposes without a thorough medical evaluation and prescription from a doctor!

Recreational cannabis contains significant amounts of THC, which is the opposite for most medical marijuana products, which generally contain little or no THC. It can still be hard to tell how much THC is in the marijuana you may be consuming!

Using arguments in favor of medicinal cannabis to promote or minimize the effects of recreational marijuana is a deceiving strategy; remember to remain critical and do your own research!

Recreational cannabis and THC Potency

- In the 1990s, average THC concentrations in cannabis were around 4%.

- Nowadays, the average concentration of THC found in recreational cannabis is around 15%, making today's cannabis much stronger and potent than it was in the past.

- This means that today's marijuana is potentially more addictive, and may be more likely to trigger negative mental effects.

- THC concentrations above 10 % are considered high, and higher concentrations of THC which are found in today's cannabis carry increased risks of addiction, depression, increased risks of psychosis, and other negative mental consequences associated with cannabis usage.

2

Cannabis & Endocannabinoid System

"Science is the father of knowledge,
but opinion breeds ignorance".

- Hippocrates

ENDOCANNABINOID SYSTEM

Cannabinoid receptors
CB-1 & CB-2

Endogenous cannabinoids
or
endocannabinoids
{Anandamide & 2-AG}

Enzymes/proteins
responsible for their
biosynthesis and
degradation

In the early weeks of a fetus development, at about 5 weeks, the endocannabinoid system can be detected. This is a system that comprise chemicals called cannabinoids, such as anandamide and 2-arachidonoylglycerol (2-AG), and receptors called cannabinoid receptors 1 and 2, to which those cannabinoids bind. Let us mention that also cannabis, which is an exogenous cannabinoid, has the ability to bind to these receptors.

Every human being has this endocannabinoid system; it is involved in the development and the well-functioning of the central nervous system including the brain and the immune system; it also helps in the regulation of other chemicals or neurotransmitters in your brain. It is involved in regulating different physiological processes such as: pain, pleasure, appetite, memory, motivation and helps in regulating the effects of cannabis in the brain.

It is important to mention that this endocannabinoid system does not need outside cannabis in order to function, it is an endogenous system with the necessary autonomy to auto stimulate itself with its endogenous cannabinoids and receptors. It does not need outside input.

When a person uses cannabis, it will bind to cannabinoid receptors and unnaturally stimulate the endocannabinoid system. For example, when a teenager uses cannabis, it might disturb the already well-established and well-functioning endocannabinoid system and prevents it from doing its naturally intended purposes, which will then interfere with the regulation of other chemicals in his or her brain and might affect the maturing or the development of that teenager's brain.

This explains why using cannabis during the critical period of brain development can have lasting disturbing consequences such as the increased risk of addiction, mental health disorders and long term cognitive dysfunctions.

ENDOCANNABINOID SYSTEM

Helps regulate other chemicals or neurotransmitters in the brain and other tissues

Participate in Homeostasis

It's a system that keeps the "Balance"

> For example: When pain goes up, endocannabinoid system is activated and endocannabinoids are released to try to reduce pain

> When anxiety goes up and cortisol increases, endocannabinoids increase as well to help reduce anxiety

The endocannabinoid system is involved in regulating:

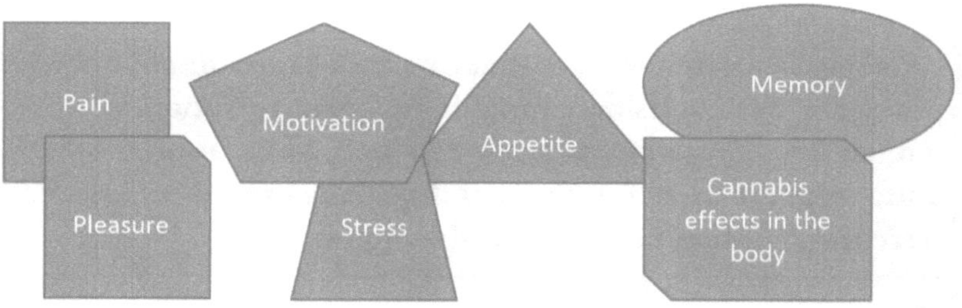

3

CBD & Medical Marijuana

"I might disagree with your opinion, but I am willing to give my life for your right to express it"

-Voltaire

CBD & MEDICAL MARIJUANA

One of the most controversial topics when it comes to cannabis is the fact that this natural plant is considered by some as a natural medicine for many conditions while others reject that notion. Praised by some and demonized by others.

But in fact, science and history shows us that cannabis has long been used in many cultures and even some ancient civilizations for recreational, medical or spiritual reasons.

The recreational use of cannabis is widespread throughout the world, and cannabis is the most used addictive substance after alcohol and tobacco. And when it comes to young people under the age of twenty-four, cannabis is the most used addictive substance among young people in North America and throughout the world.

On the other hand, sometimes recreational use can mask a form of self-treatment for anxiety, insomnia or depression. And when someone uses cannabis for self-treatment, he runs a higher risk of slipping into addiction. So we do not recommend any form of self-treatment with any substance.

Now can cannabis be used for medical reasons?

One of the chemical compounds found in cannabis is called CBD or Cannabidiol. According to current scientific knowledge, CBD is not a psychoactive substance, it is not generally used for recreational purposes because it does not provide the famous "high" sought after by recreational users of cannabis.

CBD is primarily used or studied for medical use; anti-inflammatory, antiepileptic and even antipsychotic properties have been noted in CBD.

Cannabis has been used to treat or relieve some forms of epilepsy, especially in children. Some forms of cannabis are used and are studied for the treatment of chronic pain. Other forms of cannabis or products containing cannabis are used to stimulate the appetite and reduce nausea in patients receiving chemotherapy treatments.

Research is underway to assess whether medical cannabis can be used to treat certain diseases of the immune system or the post-traumatic stress disorder in veterans of the military. It is important to note, however, that more research is needed to validate some theories around medicinal cannabis and explore other possible medical usages of cannabis.

If you're like this lady in her forties, who started using cannabis to calm her thoughts and reduce anxiety in order to get some sleep, but realized that she needed higher and higher doses of cannabis to control her anxiety, you understand that self-treatment can be dangerous and risky.

That's why I strongly advise you to stay away from any form of self-treatment with cannabis, alcohol or other substances. If you suffer from anxiety, depression, insomnia, consult a healthcare professional to properly diagnose the problem and identify the best treatment options because self-treatment is linked to the increased risk of sliding into addiction.

Main cannabinoids found in cannabis

THC	CBD
Psychoactive	Not psychoactive
Mental health risks	No known mental health risks
analgesic	antiepileptic
antiemetic	Anti-inflammatory
Appetite stimulating	Neuroprotective
	Antipsychotic

Further studies are needed to validate some practices around the medical use of cannabis.

We need to mention that there are case reports of people with different conditions who benefited from medical cannabis, especially products with high concentrations in CBD and no or low concentration in THC

Medicinal cannabis or medical marijuana is mainly used for:

- Chronic pain: conclusive evidence (especially for neuropathic pain)
- Refractory epilepsy (especially in children): growing evidence
- Spasms: spasticity in patients with multiple sclerosis: more conclusive data for oral cannabis and nabiximols than for smoked cannabis
- Nausea and vomiting (cancer, HIV / AIDS: conclusive evidence
- Loss of appetite (cancer, HIV / AIDS): conclusive evidence
- Insomnia (due to chronic pain, multiple sclerosis, fibromyalgia): moderate evidence: short- term improvement

Less evidence for the use of medicinal cannabis for:

- Chronic pain due to cancer: insufficient evidence
- Chronic pain due to fibromyalgia: few studies of good quality
- Depressive symptoms secondary to chronic pain: limited data
- Glaucoma: no studies,
- Anxiety, depression, PTSD, ADHD, autism, anorexia: no sufficient scientific evidence
- Treatment of cancer: no scientific evidence

4

What Happens When You Smoke, Inhale, Drink, or Eat Cannabis?

"Don't judge each day by the harvest you reap but
by the seeds that you plant."

—Robert Louis Stevenson

Cannabis is effective, it is fast, it has real effects on your body, your brain, your feelings and it certainly produces indisputably pleasurable effects; hence its appeal to people who choose to consume it. But consuming cannabis carries the risk of potential negative side effects, and may lead to serious consequences in some cases.

When you inhale cannabis...

When you smoke and inhale cannabis, the smoke travels to your lungs where it is absorbed into your bloodstream. It then circulates throughout your body and—most importantly—to your brain. Once there, it binds to cannabinoid receptors, stimulating the endocannabinoid system and the dopamine system in your brain. The circuitry responsible for addiction— also known as the dopamine reward system—is stimulated, causing sensations of pleasure. Cannabis also affects numerous other parts of your brain, producing a variety of reactions outlined in Table. 1- Cannabis in your brain in chapter 5. Smoking and inhaling cannabis produces rapid changes in the body and brain and its effects are felt almost immediately when consumed in this manner.

When you eat or drink cannabis...

When you eat or drink cannabis—for example, in a muffin, cake, or tea— the drug has to go through the digestive system before being absorbed into your bloodstream. Cannabis goes through the liver, where it is broken down or metabolized into other chemicals or metabolites. One chemical or metabolite produced in the liver is called 11-hydroxy-THC (11-OH- THC). This metabolite is even more potent or stronger than cannabis or THC itself. It can get you more mentally altered and its effects might last longer in your system. Therefore, when you eat or drink marijuana, the psychoactive effect takes longer to kick in—about thirty minutes or more—but the overall psychoactive effects can be increased with more loss of focus and balance, and more mental alteration than when marijuana is smoked or inhaled.

> **Edible Cannabis, when you eat or drink cannabis:**
>
> - The effects take longer to kick in: 30 minutes up to 2 hours
> - But the effects last longer: can last 8 to 12 hours
> - THC is transformed or metabolized by the liver into another chemical that is even stronger than the original THC consumed
> - And can thus do more harm
>
> **When you smoke or inhale cannabis**
>
> - The effects are felt almost immediately:
>
> The effects last: 4 to 8 hours, but can last longer for some people

5

Cannabis in Your Brain

"Turn your wounds into wisdom."

—Oprah Winfrey

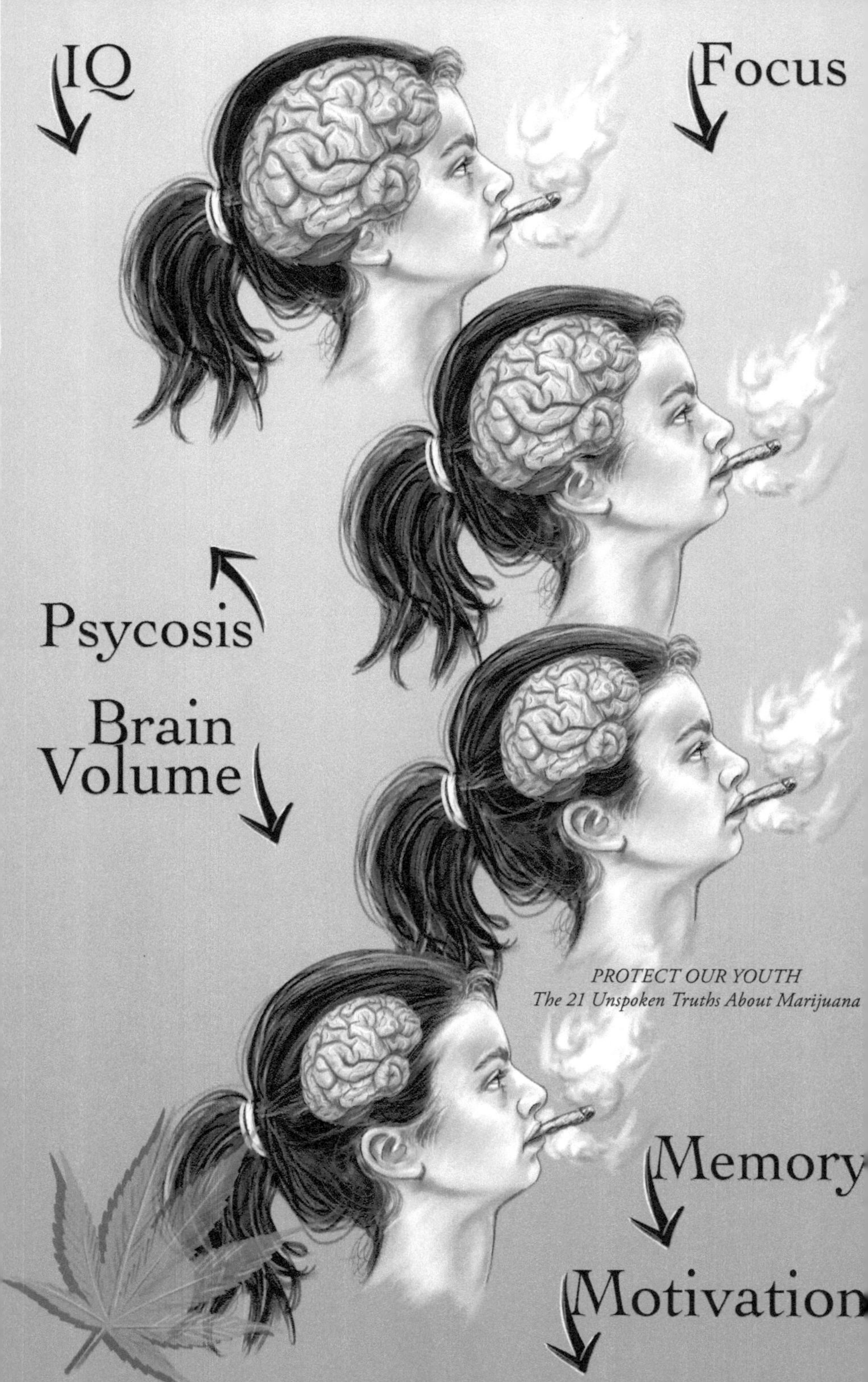
IQ
Focus
Psycosis
Brain
Volume
PROTECT OUR YOUTH
The 21 Unspoken Truths About Marijuana
Memory
Motivation

As we discussed throughout the previous chapter whether you smoke it, drink it, eat it, or inhale it, cannabis is absorbed into your blood which helps it travel to its favorite destination: your brain! Here it begins to act, either creating a 'buzz' (or a beautiful feeling), or 'getting you irrational'. It's in the delicate chemistry of the brain that marijuana acts to produce the desired—or undesirable—psychoactive effects, producing short and long-term consequences which are often hard to predict in advance.

Brain development is a very complex process; the brain starts to develop throughout the fetus' prenatal life and brain growth isn't entirely complete until around the age of twenty-five. So any physical, psychological or emotional trauma the brain experiences before the age of twenty-five is more likely to interfere with overall brain development, and is therefore more likely to cause long term damage to the brain.

Table 1 presents the different parts of the brain affected by cannabis consumption, as well as outlining some of the potential serious life consequences which could result from 'getting high'. However, it's important to acknowledge that this table is simplified, since the brain is complicated and its parts are more interconnected than can be fully outlined in any simple table! Any individual structure of the brain can be involved in controlling numerous aspects of how we behave; for example, the amygdala—one of the structures of the brain discussed in the table below—is involved both in our emotional reactions, as well as being involved in how we process memory, and in how we make decisions. Just remember that each part of the brain might also be affected by marijuana, and could subsequently affect other aspects of our behaviors not discussed below!

Table 1. How Cannabis/Marijuana Affects Your Brain

Structures of the Brain Affected by Cannabis	**Function of Brain Structure**	**Effects of cannabis**	**Potential Life consequences**
Hippocampus	Involved in memory	↓memory	↑Learning problems
Prefrontal cortex	Involved in executive functions, focus, inhibition, judgement, planning…	↓judgement, ↓concentration, ↓attention span ↓behavioral inhibition ↓executive functions	*↑Behavior problems, *↑impulsivity *↓judgment *↑risk of addiction *↑ Risk of accidents, *↓ability to learn *↑sexual impulses
Nucleus accumbens	Involved in the Reward system	Increased dopamine in the nucleus accumbens	↑addiction risk
Cerebellum	Involved in balance, movement, coordination…	Reduced balance and coordination	*↑Risk of fall, *↑Risk of accidents
Basal ganglia	Involved in movement planning and Coordination…	*slower in reacting to sudden events *↓movement planning and coordination	↑risk of car accidents
Amygdala	Involved in fear and aggressive behavior, anxiety, emotions...	If high doses of cannabis: ↑Fear ↑Anxiety ↑panic…	*Anxiety problems *panic *isolation *aggressiveness *depressive mood…
Hypothalamus	Involved in hormonal control, appetite, sleep, attachment behavior…	↑appetite and eating, ↑sleep dysregulation, ↓attachment.	*↑appetite and eating *long term sleep problems, *↑sexual impulses *↓attachment to one's family
Overall brain anatomy	-↓brain volume -thinning of the cerebral cortex -changes in cerebral white matter -in addition to the functional changes noted above [26]		

Are you under 25 years old?

Cannabis has impacts on your brain at any age, but if you're under 25 years old, your brain is still developing and will be more affected by consuming it;

You are more at risk of developing an addiction to the drug, of developing symptoms of antimotivational syndrome, learning problems, and even of developing a psychotic episode! These subjects will be discussed later in the book.

6

Cannabis: Teenagers, Young Adults

"The Strongest principle of growth lies in human choice."

—George Eliot

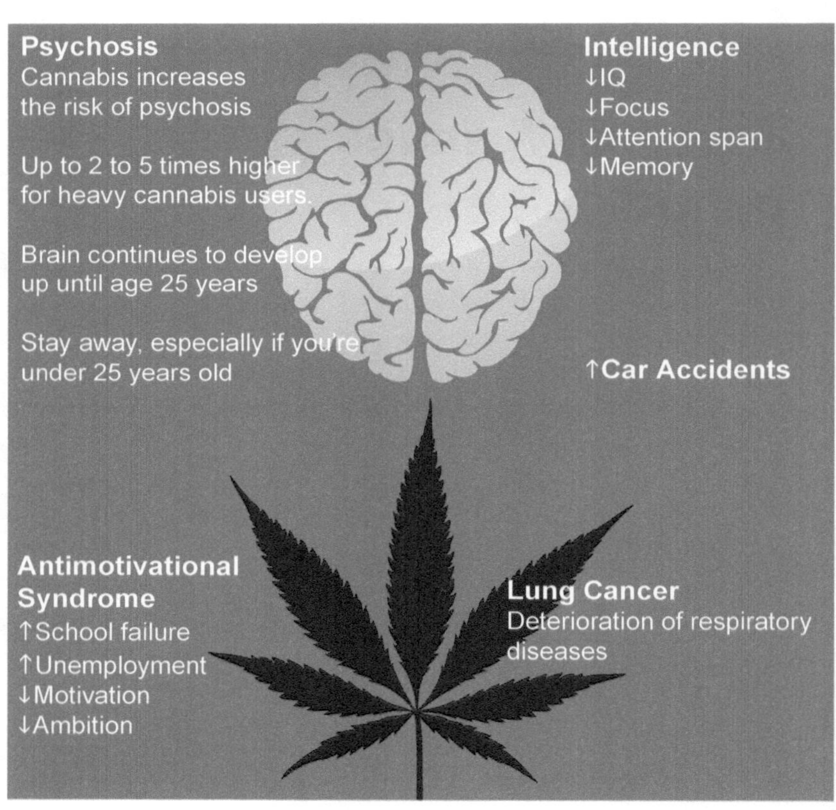

PROTECT OUR YOUTH
The 21 Unspoken Truths About Marijuana

-In our mother's womb, during the third week of fetus development, our brain begins to form…

- This process of brain development continues until around the age of twenty-five.[9,26]

-Therefore, it is extremely important to be careful with what substances the brain is exposed to during this vulnerable period, since changes to the partially developed brain can last a lifetime!

As life begins, so does the formation of the brain. Your brain starts developing in your mother's womb. At the very beginning of the fetus' third week, cells begin to clump together to begin creating what will arguably become the most crucial organ in your body, the pilot of your life, the host of your mind, the chief controller and the maestro of your organs: your brain!

This process includes the growth of different brain structures as well as the formation of crucial connections which link different parts of the brain together. It also involves the trimming of unnecessary connections over time, a process known as 'synaptic pruning'.

Your brain continues to develop and mature over the next twenty-five years. The final parts of the brain to develop are the frontal lobes; these parts are mainly involved in planning, anticipating future events, paying attention and focusing, decision making, inhibitory control, reasoning, and problem solving.

Imagine for a moment what might happen to your brain if it is exposed to a toxic substance, or to a physical or emotional trauma while it is still in the process of developing; this might slow or interfere with brain development in different ways, and might have future impacts which could be hard to predict!

> **So your thirteen-year-old or fifteen-year-old brain, or even your twenty-one-year-old brain is—unfortunately—much more vulnerable to being altered by cannabis than a forty-year-old brain would be.**

As we discuss in chapter five and chapter twelve, cannabis, especially when repetitively used by teenagers, might lead to cognitive dysfunction, difficulty controlling impulsive behaviors, reduced capacity in problem solving, reduced focus and attention and temporary drop in IQ among many other negative effects discussed in those chapters. Let us underline that these negative effects might not be fully reversible.

Also, as will be discussed in later chapters, adolescents and young adults who try cannabis are at increased risk of developing an addiction to cannabis sometime within their adult life, and are also at much higher risk of experiencing a psychotic episode as compared to adults who try marijuana.....

Stats Corner

> **Around 10% of marijuana users will slide into addiction** [10, 11, 12]
>
> **- These risks almost double for adolescents**
>
> **- About 17% of adolescents who try or use cannabis will become dependent**
>
> **- That's about 1 in 6 adolescents who will become dependent to cannabis if they try it!**
>
> **- The risk of addiction to cannabis increases between 25 to 50% for those who use it daily.**

Signs your teenager or your friend might have started using cannabis:

If you're like this mother who was wondering what's happening to his son who started to have frequent red eyes to the point that she wanted to bring him to see an optometrist, he started to eat much more food than before, he slept so much that he started missing his classes, started getting erratic behavior and was more and more rebellious and irritable, you might consider the fact that your teenager might have started using cannabis or other substances.

Some of the classic signs of cannabis usage, especially for beginners, are red eyes, an unusual exaggerated increased appetite, tiredness, increased sleep, reduced focus and attention and loss of motivation. Some people might even experience rapid heartbeat or palpitation, anxiety or panic attacks, frequent vomiting or abdominal pain, an unusual suspicious attitude or even paranoia.

7

Cannabis: Pregnancy, Breastfeeding & Sexuality

"Do what you can, with what you have,
where you are."

—Theodore Roosevelt

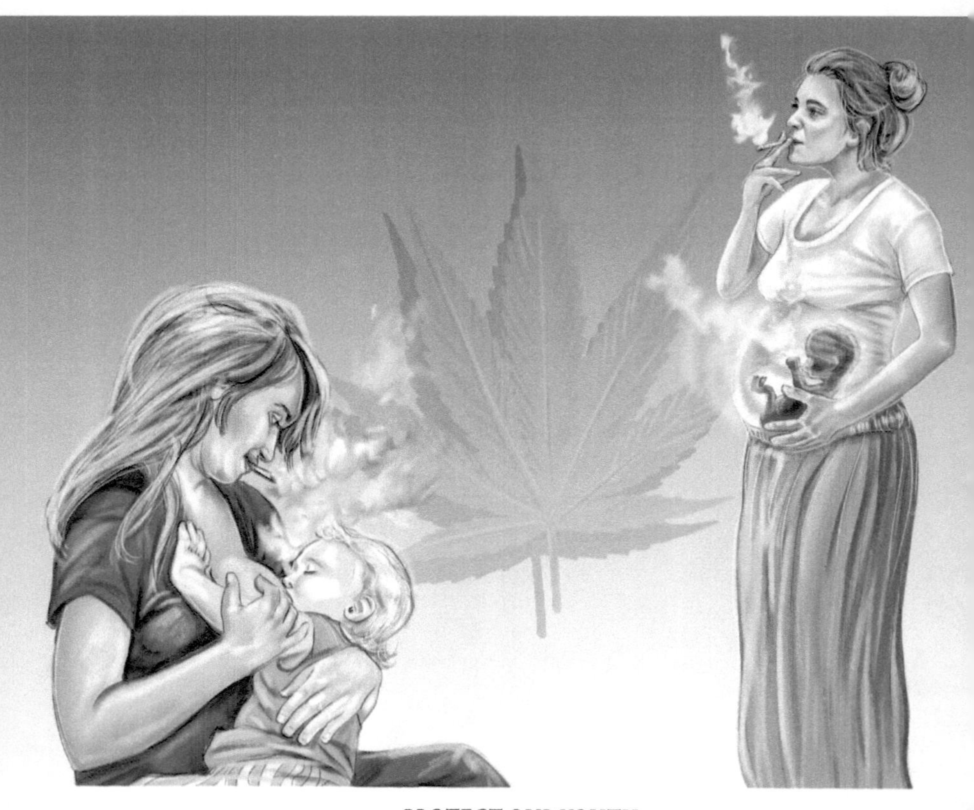

PROTECT OUR YOUTH
The 21 Unspoken Truths About Marijuana

> ***When a mother smokes, the fetus smokes, the baby smokes**
>
> **- Cannabis—specifically THC and its other cannabinoids—cross the placental barrier, so the fetus is exposed if the mother smokes, drinks, or eats cannabis products.**[13]
>
> **- The breastfed baby is also exposed to cannabis through the milk if the mother is smoking, drinking or eating cannabis products.**
>
> **- Cannabis second hand smoke, just like in tobacco, is also to be avoided.**

Cannabis, and especially THC, is known to cross the placental barrier, and about ten to thirty percent of the cannabis circulating in the mother's blood will cross into the fetus' system. Cannabis is also present in the mother's milk, so the breastfed baby may also be exposed to the drug if the mother is a marijuana user.

More research is needed to study the long term effects of using cannabis during pregnancy, but some studies have suggested that it might have lasting effects on the child's behavior throughout childhood and adolescence. Children and teenagers who were exposed to cannabis during their gestation might be more impulsive, more irritable, have difficulty with focus, attention, problem solving, anticipation and planning.[14, 15, 16]

> **CBD - Cannabidiol and Pregnancy**
>
> While CBD might not directly affect the fetus brain development, there are studies that suggest that it might increase permeability of the placenta barrier, opening the gates for other substances, toxins and medications to cross the placenta much easier and reach the fetus.[55]

Cannabis and sexuality

What we know about cannabis is certainly much less than what we don't know, especially when it comes to its effects on sexuality. We know that cannabis has been used in some cultures in the wedding night rituals to facilitate first sexual encounters between the newlyweds. Its potential ability to heighten sensory experiences, and the feeling of 'high', can be associated with increased libido, sexual impulses and encounters in some cannabis users.

However, some studies have suggested that cannabis can cause vaginal dryness and erectile dysfunction in some marijuana users. We also need to mention that since cannabis act on prefrontal cortex, it may reduce inhibition which might result in increased risk of unprotected or unsafe sex especially in teenagers.

8

Addiction Risk Factors; Who Becomes Addicted and who Does Not?

"'Tis one thing to be tempted,
another thing to fall."

—William Shakespeare

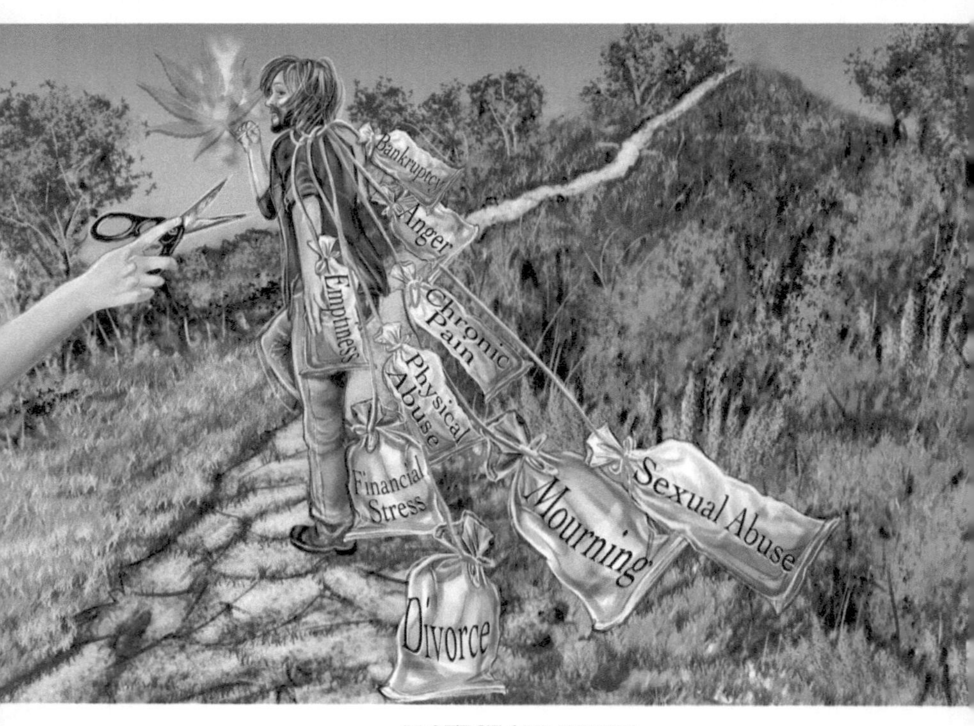

PROTECT OUR YOUTH
The 21 Unspoken Truths About Marijuana

> **When we submit to the temptation of achieving pleasure and instant gratification, it comes at a personal cost.**
>
> **When we find ourselves compromising our morals, our principles, our careers, our future goals, our families' well-being, and our health to achieve that "feel good" moment—and find ourselves doing so over and over again—here we can start talking about addiction.**

Can anyone become addicted to cannabis? Who is more at risk of succumbing to cannabis addiction? Can some people use cannabis without becoming addicted?

As you probably already know, it's in human beings' nature and design to seek out what's most pleasurable, enjoyable, and least difficult; it is only when we are following a greater purpose to achieve our goals that we choose to take a more difficult path. We all long for pleasure and the faster and easier we can obtain it, the more we risk becoming addicted to the source of pleasure. The design of the human mind allows us to experience enjoyment, but also makes us vulnerable to becoming addicted to these pleasurable experiences...

How do we biologically fall into addiction?

The Reward System or Dopamine reward pathways

Our brain is intelligently designed; the circuitry of our brain is designed to help us enjoy pleasurable activities such as great meals, good company with friends, or a stimulating encounter with a new romantic interest. The brain circuitry system responsible for allowing us to enjoy such experiences is called the Reward System or the dopamine reward pathways. These pathways in the brain encourage us to seek out these awesome, exciting, and pleasurable experiences and reinforces these types of behaviors when we seek them out, making us more likely to do so over time. Let us underscore that there are survival reasons to this reward system, food is pleasurable to encourage us to eat and stay alive, sex is pleasurable to encourage us to mate and reproduce.

You can skip the following paragraph if you're not interested in scientific explanations, but if you are, let's briefly discuss the structures of your brain which are involved in developing addictive behaviors. The reward system is first stimulated when an addictive substance or pleasurable experience is encountered; practically all addictive substances will directly or indirectly increase dopamine levels in your brain. Dopamine is a neurotransmitter or chemical in your brain that is involved in pleasure and motivation. Without going into detailed medical or scientific explanations of this circuitry, let us note that the reward system involves many parts of the brain such as the prefrontal cortex, the nucleus accumbens, the limbic system, the anterior cingulate, the ventral tegmental area, and the amygdala…

When exposed to an addictive substance, the reward circuitry stimulates some people to seek more intense experiences to achieve the same pleasure over time. As someone repetitively uses the drug, dopamine is released and over time the brain becomes 'used to' the dopamine released by the brain, it then releases less dopamine for the same amount of stimulation-or same amount of substance-over time, and therefore requires even larger amounts of stimulation to achieve the same pleasure as time progresses. Furthermore, the brain's response is dependent on numerous other factors such as genetic predisposition, morals, self-control, life stressors, protective factors, etc., and so everyone's vulnerability to addiction is based on a variety of different variables.

In these cases, the need to achieve pleasure becomes an affliction; feeling good becomes the ultimate goal, and the person can become trapped by compulsive instant gratification seeking behavior.

When we submit to the temptation of achieving pleasure and instant gratification, it comes at a personal cost.

> **When we find ourselves compromising our morals, our principles, our careers, our future goals, our families' well-being, and our health to achieve that "feel good" moment—and find ourselves doing so over and over again—here we can start seeing the signs of addiction.**

Our Brains might look similar, but each Brain is Unique!

All brains are based on a shared basic design, but they are not identical. We see variations in sizes of different brains, in the sizes of different structures of the brain, variations in the connections between different parts of the brain, and functional differences which neuroscientists can't yet fully explain or understand. Some brains are more vulnerable to addiction or mental health problems than others, for a variety of reasons. Two people from the same background, at the same age, and in comparable health could ingest the same drug, and while one will be fine, the other could experience a psychotic episode! We are all unique, and due to a host of genetic, emotional, and nurturing differences, we might all be affected in unique ways if we choose to use drugs.

<u>Who gets addicted and Who does not?</u>

Stats Corner

Not all drugs or alcohol users become addicted

- About 10% to 20% of all substance users will lose control and slide into addiction [17]

- 50% of the risk of substance addiction can be attributed to genetic factors [17]

- Additional risk factors are involved in triggering the addiction, if the user is exposed to addictive substances.

- Teenagers and Young Adults are at higher risk of becoming addicted to cannabis

So the question is: can anyone become addicted to cannabis or other drugs? The tricky answer is both "yes" and "no". Given the right circumstances, the right substances, the right experiences, and the right timing, I believe anyone can develop an addiction of some kind. Some might become addicted to cannabis, others to cocaine, alcohol, or amphetamines. Others still to pornography, internet usage, cellphones or social media, videogames, or to watching sports. Those who are vulnerable, like the high sensation seekers or novelty-seekers, are at increased risk whenever they engage in thrill-seeking or pleasure-seeking behaviors which expose them to the possibility of becoming addicted.

Some studies suggest that about 10% to 20% percent of substance users will become addicted to the substances they consume.[17] Genetics plays a major role in determining who will or won't become addicted to substances, and researchers suggest up to 50% of this risk is determined by your genetic predisposition to addictive behaviors in the first place.[17]

Many other risk factors also play a role, such as life stressors, family history, brain developmental stage and age, and the type of drugs being consumed. Teenagers are far more vulnerable to developing an addiction when they try an addictive substance than adults are.

Addiction Risk Factors

Table 2.

Do you have a parent, sibling, or relative who has struggled with a drug or alcohol addiction?
Are you addicted to alcohol or other substances right now, or do you feel you've shown addictive behaviors in the past?
Are you going through a tough time in your life?
Do you feel emotionally fragile or vulnerable at this moment?
Are you hanging around people who are using cannabis or other drugs, or do you have easy access to drugs?
Are you suffering from anxiety or depression?
Are your parents going through a separation or divorce? Are you going through a break up or divorce yourself? Do you feel you've had a traumatic childhood?
Have you experienced physical, sexual, or psychological abuse in the past?
Are you under financial stress, or having a difficult time making ends meet?
Are you experiencing conflicts at home?
Would you describe your family as being dysfunctional? Are you a teenager or young adult?
Do you have a diagnosis of Attention Deficit and Hyperactivity Disorder (ADHD), or suspect that you might have the condition?
Are you suffering from a personality disorder?
Are you suffering from a psychotic disorder?
Do you often gamble, or find it hard to stop gambling when you start in the first place?
Have you recently lost your job, or have you been experiencing stress and conflict in the workplace?

If you said "yes" to any of the questions above, you may be at increased risk of abusive or addictive usage of cannabis, alcohol, or other drugs. But even if you answered "no" to all of these questions, this doesn't completely eliminate your risk, since it's difficult to predict how any individual might react to taking drugs for the first time!

One way or the other, these questions highlight some of the major risk factors which distinguish "social" users of cannabis from those who tend to fall into drug abuse and dependence. Having one or more of these risk factors does not imply that you are doomed to develop an addiction, it simply means that the statistical risk is increased. For example, if your father had a drug addiction problem, it's statistically more likely that you would develop a drug problem as well, but it does not necessarily mean that you are condemned to that problem yourself !

Family History: A Big Risk Factor

> **We have zero control on the family we are born into, we do not chose our genetic makeup, or our biology.**
>
> **We not only inherit our genes from our family, but we also learn our habits, our understanding of life, and of the ways to cope with challenges and obstacles we face.**
>
> **But, we are not condemned to live our lives like they did!**

As stated previously, fifty percent of the risk of developing an addiction can be attributed to your genetic background. But fortunately, we are made up of more than just our genes! Generally, additional risk factors also play a role; it takes cumulative biological, environmental, and psychosocial factors to trigger an addiction.

In addition to genetic predisposition to addictive behaviors, we also have a tendency to repeat what we know, what we see, and what's been around us during our formative years. If you grow up with abusive drug use in your environment, you're more likely to re-enact the same behaviors.

The tough reality is that we cannot choose our family, we cannot decide where we are born or where we grow up. We aren't free to choose our family background. This means we face a bigger mountain to climb, a bigger challenge to overcome when raised within a dysfunctional family or a family marred by substance abuse. If this is your situation, you may wish to avoid addictive substances altogether since you face a greater risk of becoming addicted should you choose to try them. If you have a family history of alcohol or drug abuse—meaning a parent, brother, sister, cousin, uncle or aunt, or grandparent abused these substances—I suggest you avoid addictive substances such as cannabis because of the increased risk of developing an addiction yourself.

> **There is a bigger mountain to climb, a bigger challenge to overcome, a larger wave to surf when you come from a dysfunctional family or a family marred by substance abuse. But you can still overcome.**

Trauma in your past?

If you've gone through traumatic life experiences in your past such as verbal, physical, or sexual abuse, your ability to regulate your emotions might be weakened, your stress coping mechanisms might be shaky, the ability to cope with stress is fragile, the real trust in people might be broken, your choices might be compromised, the fear can be deafening and the self-confidence might be sleeping. If you combine this psychological risk factors with social, biological and environmental risk factors, the risk of falling into addiction might be greatly increased…. Be aware, and take care!

Life stressors

During stressful life circumstances, a stress hormone called cortisol increases in your brain and body, It might be tempting to consider using drugs such as cannabis to provide temporary relief and ''feel good'' moments during particularly challenging times. However, the temporary relief drugs might bring us can easily become a sensation we begin to miss and return to experience over and over again. By seeking respite from stressful life events, we might unwittingly find ourselves slipping into drug abuse.

It's important to note that not all those who try drugs will become addicted; only ten to twenty percent of drugs users will lose control and fall into drug abuse or dependence. Science still can't fully explain why some people remain in control of their drug use, but we know that biogenetic factors, psychological factors, social and environmental stressors, life development stage, and family history all play a role.[17]

Table 3: Biological, Psychosocial, and Environmental Risk Factors for Developing a Drug Dependence

Biological Risk Factors	- Genetic predisposition - Stage of development of your brain (ex. adolescent, young adult) - Medical condition (ex. Chronic pain,..) - Psychiatric conditions (depression, anxiety, psychotic disorders, schizophrenia, bipolar disorder), personality disorders, ADHD,..) - Abuse of other substances
Risk factors related to a history of trauma	- Physical abuse victim - Sexual abuse victim - Psychological abuse victim - Bullying victim
Social-Environmental risk factors	- Experiencing divorce, Separation, or relationship break-up or are the Child of Parents going through a divorce or separation - Experiencing peer pressure - Experiencing economic stress - Experiencing stressful life events (ex. New job, new relationship, wedding),…. - Group of friends or close relatives who use drugs - Easy access to the drug - Judicial or employment problems - Chaotic home life - Grieving the loss of a loved one… -Growing up with a feeling of rejection -Growing up fatherless or motherless

9

How Do You Know You're Sliding from Cannabis Use Into Abuse?

"You may have to fight a battle more than once, to win it."

—Margaret Thatcher

Stats Corner

> **- Around 10% of marijuana users will slide into addiction** [10, 11, 12 54]
>
> **-These risks almost double for teenagers**
>
> **- About 17 % or 1 in 6 teenagers who try cannabis will slide into addiction.**
>
> **-Note that cannabis is not the only addictive drug out there; the risk of becoming addicted to alcohol is about 15%, tobacco/nicotine (33%), heroine (23%), and cocaine (17%).**
>
> **- Still, it's important to consider the potential addictive properties of cannabis as well, especially given the fact that for teenagers and regular users, the risks are often worse!**
>
> **- Remember, the risks of developing a dependence on cannabis jump to 25-50% for those who use marijuana on a daily basis!**

Quick reflection Questions

Are you consuming more cannabis than you intended to?

Are you consuming cannabis more frequently?

Are you hiding your drug use from your loved ones?

Are you having conflicts with your family or friends about your drug use?

Are you lying about your substance use?

Are you having financial problems because of your drug use? Are you neglecting your responsibilities due to your drug use?

Are you neglecting family relationships or close friends?

Are you prioritizing peers who share your habit and neglecting other meaningful social interactions?

If you answered "yes" to any of the above questions, you may be at increased risk of abusing cannabis—or have potentially already fallen into that category! Many people who are becoming addicted or are regularly abusing drugs might still be in denial about their actions; you may not share others' views about the dangers and risks associated with your own drug consumption or your behaviors when using drugs. Do you ever find yourself getting into heated discussions or conflicts with loved ones, or accuse them of exaggerating when it comes to the frequency of your drug use?

When you start receiving criticism from the people close to you about your use of addictive substances, when you start experiencing guilt or shame, when you find yourself unable to control the quantity you consume or when you start taking more than you intended to, when you're tempted to lie to your friends or family about your substance use, when you experience withdrawal symptoms on those occasions when you choose to refrain, when you start to ignore meaningful social interactions because you're either focused on finding the drug or hanging out with peers who share your habit, when you start to ignore your usual responsibilities or activities or start needing the drug to be able to sleep or relax, then you know you are probably sinking into marijuana abuse or addiction.

10

A Gateway Drug-A Front Door Drug?

Can Marijuana Use Lead to The Abuse of Other Drugs?

> "A journey of a thousand miles begins
> with a single step."
>
> **—Lao Tzu**

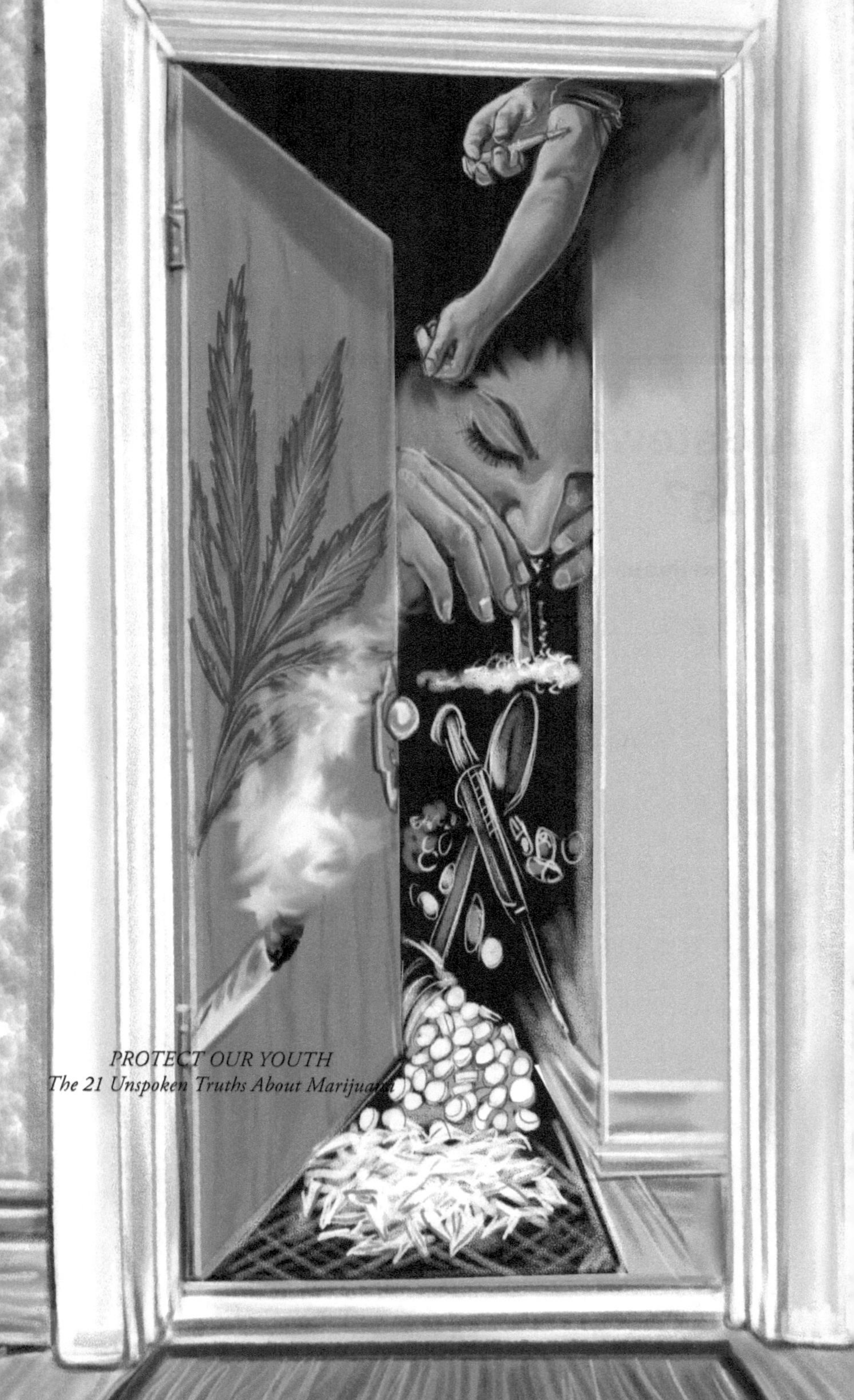
PROTECT OUR YOUTH
The 21 Unspoken Truths About Marijuana

Marijuana, a gateway drug? A Front Door drug?

-If you use marijuana, especially during adolescent years or as a young adult, you have an increased risk of developing addictions to other illicit drugs later in life. [18, 19, 20, 21]

-It's also true for other drugs, including alcohol and tobacco,

-The addiction to any substance is associated with a higher statistical risk of falling into addiction to other substances or illicit drugs. [18, 19, 20, 21]

The use of cannabis during vulnerable stages of brain development can lead to changes to your endocannabinoid system, and consequently cause changes to your dopamine reward pathway. Additionally, it could interfere with the maturing process of other crucial parts of the brain involved in behavior inhibition and decision, such as the prefrontal cortex. These brain chemistry changes contribute to increasing the risks for teenagers and young adults who are exposed to cannabis to seeking more powerful psychoactive drugs throughout their lifetime.

While the majority of cannabis users might not abuse other drugs later on, researchers have noticed that those who use cannabis as teenagers are at higher statistical risk of developing drug dependency behaviors with other drugs later in life; [18, 19, 20, 21] this tendency is what some people are referring to when they call cannabis "a gateway drug". For example, those addicted to cannabis are three times more likely to fall into heroin addiction later in life. It's important however to clarify that this tendency is also true of all other drugs, not just marijuana; the abuse of any substance—including alcohol and tobacco—is associated with increased risks of developing other substance addictions.

11

Cannabis & Opioid Crisis

"It is better to light one candle than
to curse the darkness."

- Chinese Proverb

Cannabis and Opioid Crisis

The opioid crisis is a sad, tragic and unfortunate situation and for those people who are going through opioid use disorder or dependence, I command your courage to fight for a better day. Keep on the fight, we are with you and we do support your winnable fight. I believe that, as a society, we are called to support you, not only with our kind words for political or ideological purposes, but with more research, more understanding and more solutions.

Head on, a difference needs to be made between using medicinal cannabis to treat pain, which is an important topic to explore, versus using cannabis to treat an already existing opioid addiction, which I believe is not a viable strategy.

So if medicinal cannabis, I highlight 'medicinal', can be one of the solutions to treat pain, let's do more research, let's dig more and see whether cannabis can really be one of the many other non-opioid classic painkillers. I advise against trying to self-medicate with recreational marijuana for pain or other medical conditions.

However, trying to fight an opioid addiction with THC-based cannabis might be doomed for failure, because people will probably soon or later come back to opioids. This would be like trying to treat an alcoholic by giving him valium, xanax or other benzodiazepines such as ativan, clonazepam for long term use, you're guaranteed that the alcoholic will certainly develop an addiction to valium or other benzodiazepines and might later come back to alcohol. The same reality applies to cannabis and opioids

> ### *Crosstalk*
>
> **-There is a bidirectional communication between the opioid system and the cannabinoid system in your body, a phenomenon called Crosstalk, that will increase the risk of going back and forth from one substance to the other**
>
> **-If you try to treat opioid addiction with THC-cannabis, you might get a temporary relief from opioids, but due to crosstalk, you will most probably end up going back to opioids later on.**

Opioids are powerful pain killers that are supposedly prescribed by healthcare professionals for severe pain that cannot evidently be controlled by other non-opioid medications. Yes, opioids are highly addictive, they activate the circuitry in your brain, known as the Reward System, which reinforces pleasure. We need to mention that while cannabis activate the same circuitry and can also result into addiction for some people, opioids are more addictive than cannabis. After a certain time, tolerance develops and opioid users need higher and higher dosages to either reduce pain or to feel pleasure, and this tolerance might lead to overdose that can result in deaths. Patients usually start with prescribed opioids and some will end up on more powerful opioids such as heroin or unsupervised fentanyl.

Does Alcohol or cannabis addictions increase the risk of heroin addiction?

As I mentioned above, Opioids, especially the powerfully addictive heroin, are far more addictive than cannabis, but cannabis, especially recreational cannabis with high concentrations of THC can lead into addiction for about 10% recreational users, and an addiction to any substance increases the risk of sliding into addictions to other substances.

According to the US National Survey on Drug Use and Health, most people who are addicted to heroin have been addicted to at least one other substance before, most of the time, alcohol, cannabis, cocaine or other opioids; People who are addicted to alcohol are two times more likely to become addicted to heroin, those addicted to marijuana are three times more likely to become addicted to heroin, those addicted to cocaine are fifteen times more likely to be addicted to heroin and those with an addiction to prescription opioid painkillers are forty times more likely to become addicted to heroin sometime in their life.

> - **People who are addicted to alcohol are 2 times more likely to become addicted to heroin,**
>
> - **Those addicted to marijuana are 3 times more likely to become addicted to heroin sometime in their life.**

As for the debate about whether cannabis can be used to reduce opioid usage for the treatment of pain, I advise more research so that we can have educated opinions and be able to offer evidence-based treatments with rigorous scientific evidences.

Let us not make this an ideological, political or economic debate, let us instead face it scientifically in a neutral way, let us approach this as a health issue, not a political or ideological issue so that we can avoid premature and unfounded conclusions on either side of the argument.

While we continue to forcefully reinforce the evidence-based strategies that we already have in place to face the opioid crisis, naloxone, methadone, buprenorphine, needle exchanges; we need to remain open and do more research in case we have a dormant unexploited treatment that we can improve for the common good of our fellow citizens.

> - **Trying to treat an opioid addiction with THC-based Cannabis, is like trying to treat an alcoholic with a long term use of Valium, Xanax or ativan.**
> - **This will temporarily reduce alcohol while the person is developing a new addiction to Xanax or valium or other benzodiazepine, and finally they will possibly come back to alcohol later. The same principle applies to cannabis and opioids.**

12

Can Cannabis Lead To Intellectual Decline or Cognitive Dysfunction?

"There are those that look at things the way they
are, and ask why? I dream of things that never
were, and ask why not?"

—Robert F. Kennedy

From table 1: How cannabis/marijuana affects your brain

Structures of the Brain Affected by Cannabis	**Function of Brain Structure**	**Effects of cannabis**	**Potential Life consequences**
Hippocampus	Involved in memory	↓memory	↑Learning problems
Prefrontal cortex	Involved in executive functions, focus, inhibition, judgement, planning…	↓judgement, ↓concentration, ↓attention span ↓behavioral inhibition ↓executive functions	*↑Behavior problems, *↑impulsivity *↓judgment *↑risk of addiction *↑Risk of accidents, *↓ability to learn *↑sexual impulses

As discussed in chapter 5, marijuana affects different parts of your brain; memory is temporarily affected and chronic use can even affect the hippocampus, which is one of the main structures of the brain involved in memory retention. Cannabis also affects the prefrontal cortex, involved in behavior inhibition, focus, attention, planning, organization and anticipation; potential long term effects on these brain areas associated with chronic marijuana usage can lead to learning problems, academic or even professional failures. In fact, regular cannabis users can see their I.Q score drop almost 10 points! Some studies have disputed these findings since they didn't find significant loss in IQ points for early cannabis users. We need to note that cognitive effects of marijuana might not be fully reversible once marijuana consumption ceases.

- **For some heavy and regular adolescent cannabis users, I.Q score might drop almost 10 points,** [22]

- **For some teenagers, this might not be reversible even when they stop consuming cannabis during adulthood.** [22, 63]

13

Antimotivational Syndrome:
can cannabis kill my career, my ambitions &
my dreams?

> "Courage is like a muscle;
> it is strengthened by use"
>
> **—Ruth Gordon**

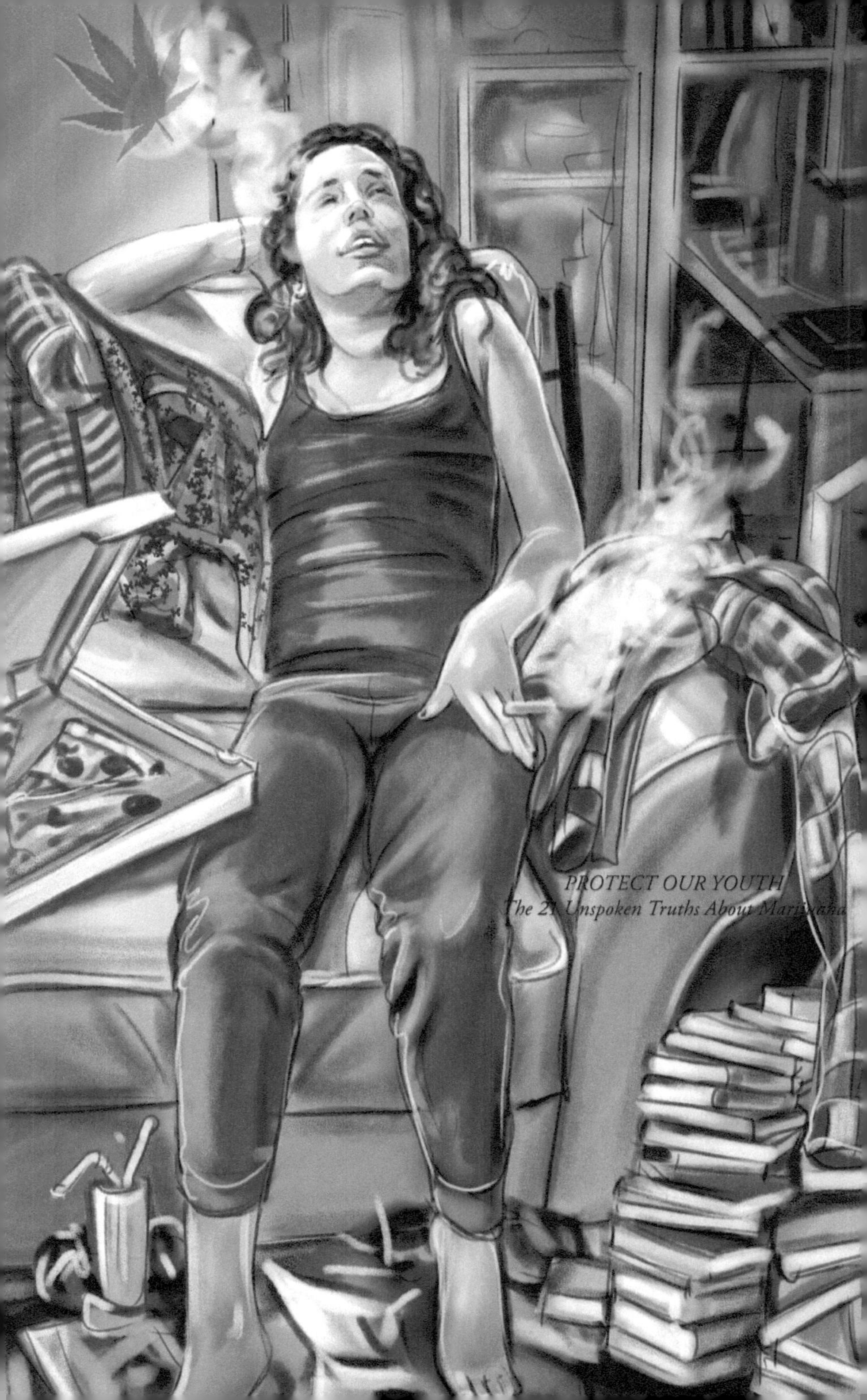
PROTECT OUR YOUTH
The 21 Unspoken Truths About Marijuana

> **For some cannabis and substance abusers the motivation towards pleasure-seeking and instant gratification sometimes overtakes the real motivation towards a more ambitious, fulfilling, balanced and goal-oriented life.**
>
> **When addiction takes over, soon the "high life" replaces the real life! The feck life becomes the life.**

Picture an eighteen-year-old student, a great guy with a positive attitude who is highly motivated, ambitious, and intelligent. This student is both academically and socially active, is close to his mother, and is very helpful in pitching in around the house with any necessary domestic chores.

Little by little, this portrait of him starts to change; he begins getting into more frequent conflicts with his mom, loses interest towards getting good grades, spends less time with his family and increasing amounts of time outside the home. He no longer wants to set challenging goals for himself anymore, and all his ambitious life-plans start to go downhill. He makes new friends—mainly toxic friends, whom his mother disapproves of—and his childhood best friends are shown the door, one by one.

His ultimate goal becomes instant gratification; he spends his time listening to music, smoking "weed", chilling with friends, and telling each other stories in noisy smoke-filled apartments and bars. Our student's need for pleasure overtakes his motivation to live a more fulfilling, balanced, ambitious, and goal-oriented life. The "high life" replaces real life…

> **This lifestyle of drug use associated with a shift in personal goals, this lethargy, this loss of motivation, this lack of ambition and purpose, this neglect of priorities, this apathy is what is commonly described by health professionals as "Antimotivational Syndrome".**

This syndrome is one of the most common side effects associated with chronic cannabis usage, one which is shared with almost all other addictions as well. When taken regularly, cannabis has serious impacts on your level of motivation and often traps users in a cycle of lethargy and apathy which can last for months or years at a time, without accessing the proper help.

Cannabis, especially when it slides into dependence or addiction, can absolutely distract you from thinking about your ambitions, and leave your dreams by the wayside. Chronic marijuana consumption creates its own selfish meaning in your life; it starts scheduling regular appointments with you on a daily basis, and soon you start looking forward to that beautiful relaxation time you are spending with your weed every day at the expense of everything else you used to find important.

Smoking a joint or "vaping weed" becomes the best moment of your day, and spending time thinking about your goals, ambitions, and dreams becomes optional. Spending time with your marijuana-using friends rises to the top of your priority list, while spending time with your family and caring friends falls to the bottom of the list. Real friends, real family, real goals, and real dreams suddenly are perceived to be boring. Making jokes with fake and superficial friends while smoking marijuana takes precedence over all else, while the people who care about you the most begin to increasingly worry about your well-being.

> **Over the longer term, antimotivational syndrome often leads to a dysfunctional and deficient lifestyle. Professional, academic, and social failures keep piling up, feelings of self-worth and confidence decrease, and depression starts knocking on the door.**

While the symptoms of antimotivational syndrome are often mistaken for those of depression, they are both separate mental health conditions. However, the consequences of losing one's interest in previously loved activities and ceasing to engage in meaningful social interactions and relationships often leads to symptoms of depression over the longer term. So it's worth knowing how to detect antimotivational syndrome if you begin to recognize its negative consequences in your own behavior, since they can sometimes lead us down a path of lifestyle choices which might be impossible to reverse.

> **Prolonged and important use of cannabis may decrease dopamine synthesis in areas of the brain called striatum, and this is one of the possible scientific explanations for the development of antimotivational syndrome in prolonged users of cannabis and other addictive substances.**
>
> **Note also the possibility of serotonin decrease for heavy and chronic cannabis users; this could be an additional explanation for the antimotivational syndrome or even increased risk of depression.**

14

Cannabis: Social Life and Family Relationships

"When wealth is lost, nothing is lost. When health is lost, something is lost. When character is lost, everything is lost."

—Billy Graham

> **When overwhelmed by drug addiction, sadly**
>
> - **what's easy becomes the goal, what's immediate becomes the focus, what's feck becomes cool, the quick pleasure becomes the aim, immediate gratification becomes the purpose.**
> - **What's lasting becomes optional, what's hard becomes annoying, what's real becomes uncool, what's worthy becomes tasteless and what's long becomes pointless.**

Can cannabis negatively affect your relationships?

Before going any further in this discussion, it will be useful to keep in mind that there is a difference between a social life based on obtaining pleasure versus one which is based on principals and achieving fulfillment.

You can socialize often, be surrounded constantly by others, yet still feel lonely; you can have numerous people in your life, yet still feel isolated!

This may seem like a contradictory statement, but it speaks to a truth which I observe every day in my profession as a psychiatrist. There are people who spend their teenage years, their twenties, or even their middle age wasting so much of their valuable time nurturing superficial relationships focused around achieving pleasure and simple gratification. These individuals surround themselves with many frivolous friends, and involve themselves in numerous activities, yet forgot to nurture long-lasting relationships that truly matter. They focus so intently on pleasurable activities that they forget the true meaning of happiness, which is the attainment of a well- balanced life.

> **We can socialize a lot, be with people a lot, be surrounded a lot, yet still feel lonely. We can have numerous people in our life, yet still feel isolated.**

Getting back to the subject of marijuana, using the drug can certainly provide relief for some people, may cause physically pleasurable sensations (and potentially lead to the occasional laughing fit), but it would be difficult to say that it necessarily leads to a permanent state of fulfillment or happiness. The pleasurable feelings associated with marijuana can be very sneaky, since when ingesting marijuana becomes a person's ultimate goal the person will sometimes end up resorting to deceptive behavior to maintain their habit, like lying to the family or partner, misusing family finances, sometimes stealing, neglecting family and personal priorities and so forth. This priority shift was discussed in the chapter on antimotivational syndrome.

Some people argue that cannabis has the capacity to increase social interactions with friends but neglect to mention the type and quality of increased social interactions; yes, it may increase pleasure of being within a social group, the desire to spend more time with peers who share the same habits, but it may also distance you from those friends who disagree with your drug consumption behavior, and potentially isolate you from those who attempt to get you back on the road towards achieving your dreams.

> **- Cannabis abuse or dependence may decrease the pleasure you feel spending sober time with your family, and with your ambitious and goal oriented friends.**
>
> **- It may increase your desire for pleasurable, yet superficial, impermanent social interactions, and decrease your interest in nurturing long lasting social ties based in sobriety.**
>
> **- These social tendencies are observed in the social relationships of almost all people suffering from substance addictions!**

15

Peer Pressure

"When you say 'Yes' to others, make sure you are
not saying 'No' to yourself."

—Paolo Coelho

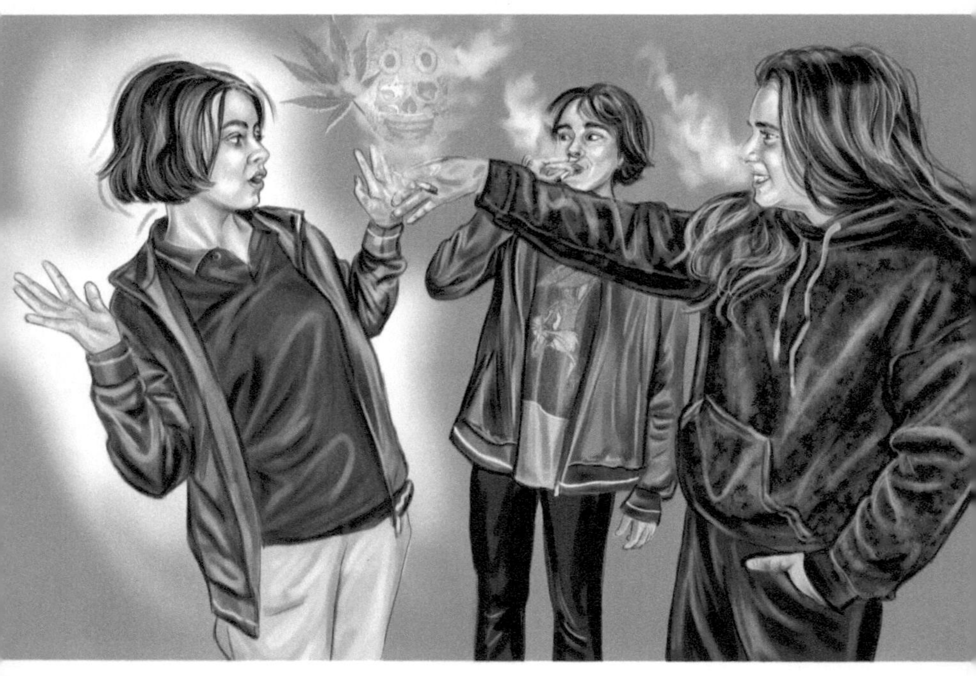

PROTECT OUR YOUTH
The 21 Unspoken Truths About Marijuana

Stats Corner

> **- Cannabis is the most commonly used addictive drug after tobacco and alcohol** [24]
>
> **- The rate of adolescents' and young adults'(15-24) cannabis usage is 2 times higher than that of adults 25 years and older** [5]
>
> **- 22.5 million Americans have used cannabis within the previous month based on a 2015 national survey** [2]

While it's comforting to feel we belong somewhere, and it's clear that loneliness, rejection, solitude, and difficulty making friends are painful experiences, the neediness and desperation with which we seek feelings of acceptance and love can sometimes lead us to accept very high personal costs.

Consider the case of a certain fourteen-year-old girl, rejected and abandoned by her dad, psychologically abused by her mother, and sexually abused by numerous of her mother's boyfriends. Feelings of loneliness are practically inscribed on an invisible sign hanging around her neck! Without friends, she's been moving more than twice a year with her mother for many years; she has been rejected and bullied so badly, that she's been forced to switch schools four times since having started secondary school two years ago. She feels alone at home and at school, and desperately needs to be accepted at all costs.

She is invited by a cool group of older schoolmates to join their table, and she feels accepted and taken care of; for the first time since having started high school, she no longer feels afraid of being bullied, and she begins to spend as much time as possible with her new friends, much of which is spent smoking marijuana. Her new gang becomes a part of her everyday life and she has a lot of fun, but it's not all positive; she also experiences a lot of hurt along the way. She begins to realize that her acceptance in the group is conditional on continuing to behave like the group, talk like the group, share the same lifestyle as the group, and dress like her friends. In becoming like the group, she is not free to totally be herself. She cannot make her own decisions, dress as she wishes, or think for herself; she finds the group's acceptance and affection is entirely conditional on behaving as they wish.

Compromising her basic principles becomes her new norm; the more she compromises, the more she smokes marijuana, the more her judgement is affected, and the more lost she becomes. Depression sets in, and she begins to set fewer goals for herself, and the more suicidal she becomes as the years pass.

Submitting to peer pressure to seek acceptance, affection, or because of fear comes with a very big price. The big question you should ask yourself: is it worth the cost? Surrendering to peer pressure might cost you your positive relationships with your family members, your real friends, your financial savings, and your health or ultimately even your life!

When all is said and done it's okay to accept risks in life, but before you make the decision to make using drugs a part of your life, ask yourself again: am I more vulnerable? Am I at higher risk of addiction or psychosis? If so, is it worth the risk? Once you've done this, go ahead and decide what's best for you knowing that you've looked at the situation clearly.

- Is it worth risking developing an addiction, is it worth risking your family, your real friends, is it worth risking psychosis, depression, or even suicide just to be accepted, just to fit in, just to please those friends who will not be around a few years from now? Is it worth the possible price?

- If you're an adolescent you're at increased risk of surrendering to peer pressure and you are more suggestible than the adults are

If you use Cannabis, especially during adolescent years or as a young adult, you have an increased risk of developing addictions to other illicit drugs later in life.[18,19,20,21]

16

Cannabis – Depression – Anxiety

Can using Cannabis lead to Symptoms of Depression and Anxiety?

"Be kind, for everyone you meet is
fighting a harder battle."

—Plato

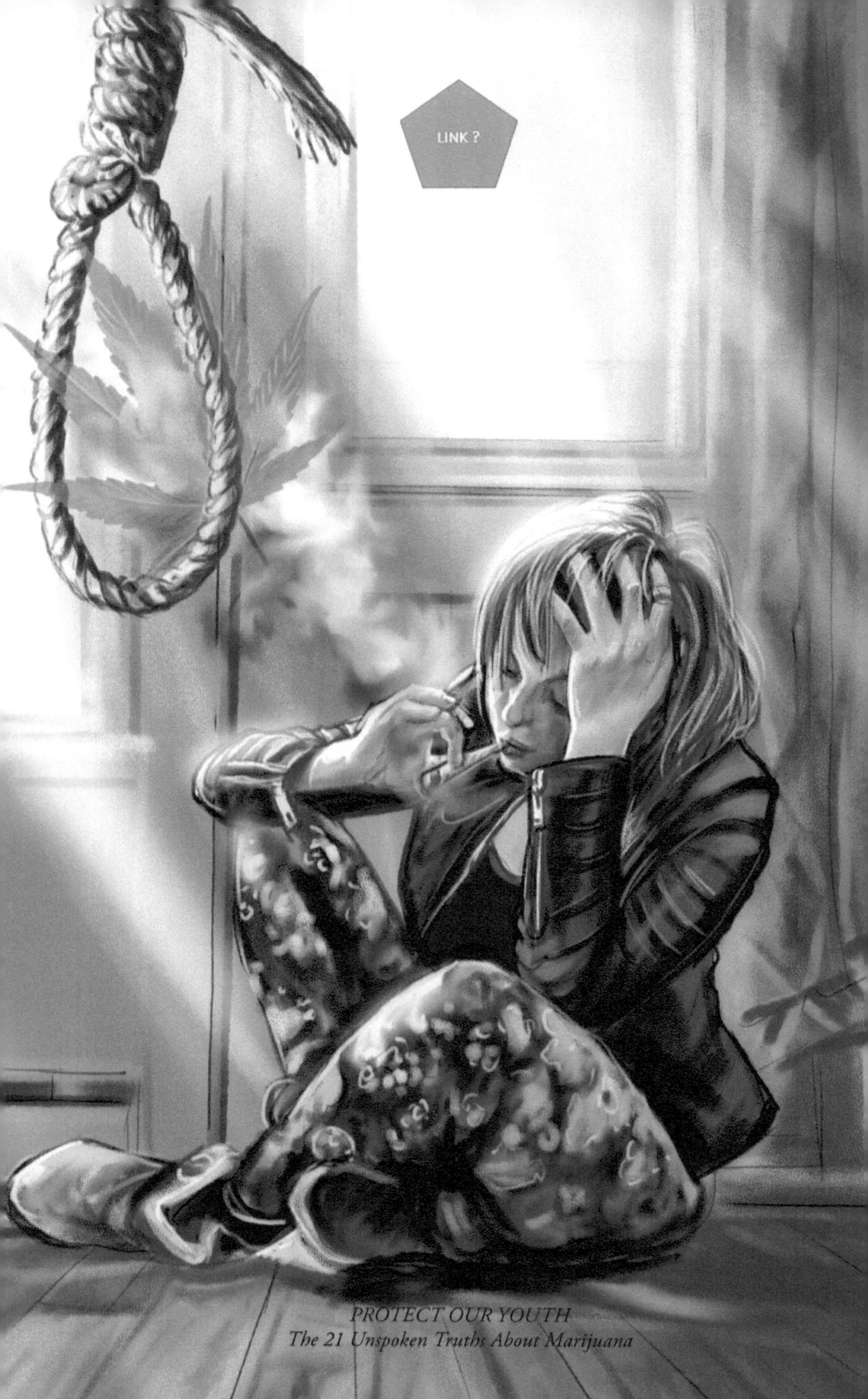

LINK ?
PROTECT OUR YOUTH
The 21 Unspoken Truths About Marijuana

> **Marijuana can make you feel good in the moment, but that longed for 'feel-good moment' can play tricks on us;**
>
> **When use turns to abuse, marijuana could be a 'smoke-screen' hiding our profound suffering and pain, symptoms that will only become obvious to us later on down the road of life.**

One of the reasons marijuana is popular and is so commonly used by adolescents and by young adults is that it makes some people feel good, in fact, very good. It can certainly decrease anxiety for some time, and some even use it on a daily basis before going to bed, as they feel they can't sleep without its beautiful powers of relaxation. But is there anything else hidden behind that beautiful feeling? Is it a great gift from nature, or could it be a rose with thorns?

> **- Cannabis usage, especially in teenagers, is associated with increased risks of depression** [45-53]
>
> **- Cannabis users, especially daily and heavy users, are 2 to 4 times more likely to experience depressive symptoms later in life than non-cannabis users.**
>
> **- Significant quantities of cannabis affect those parts of your brain—like the amygdala—which regulate anxiety, fear, and emotions.**
>
> **- For some users, cannabis can cause symptoms of anxiety or paranoia, and may even result in panic attacks or symptoms of depression.**
>
> **- Significant amounts of marijuana THC has been shown to reduce serotonin activity in the brain, which has been associated with increased risks of depression.**

Neglecting the Cornerstones

When we fall into an addiction of any kind, there is a tendency to neglect certain aspects of our lives, and sometimes crucial cornerstones are carelessly set aside. But we can be all-but-certain that those ignored pieces will be missing later on down the line when we will be needing them the most!

We can choose to seek immediate gratification through marijuana, we can enjoy superficial relief from our problems and negative feelings, we can hang out with superficial people and ignore major pieces of the puzzle like family, work, physical exercise, and significant relationships. But when we are finally reminded of what we've been missing—as we fall back to the reality of solid ground—we are eventually forced to confront the consequences which accompany the easy choices and quick fixes we chose to make earlier on.

When you realize that you've been living in a static way—enjoying the moment, but not advancing anywhere, while everyone else has kept progressing—regrets begin to arise and you may start to blame either your own behavior, circumstances beyond your control, or the people who surround you. Anxiety starts settling in, as do worries, and regrets about missed past opportunities. When we realize we have few realistic prospects for future opportunities, depression starts knocking at the door, and then it enters and makes itself at home!

> **When use turns into abuse, you take drugs to diffuse the emotional pain, but the more you take, the more anxious you become. The more anxious you become, the more you take to try to ease the pain, yet become even less functional and experience even more emotional pain.**
>
> **You return to marijuana, alcohol or other drugs again and again for the 'buzz' you need to freeze this pain, but only end up leading yourself down the path of an ever deepening cycle filled with antimotivational syndrome, professional failures, regrets, and symptoms of depression.**

Additionally, it's important to remember that cannabis affects many parts of your brain simultaneously, including the amygdala which is the part of the brain involved in the regulation of our emotions. When you consume large quantities of cannabis, the amygdala is affected and you may subsequently experience symptoms of fear or anxiety, or even panic attacks. If you have a family history of depression or anxiety, feel you are suffering from a drug or alcohol addiction, if you are a teenager or young adult under the age of twenty- five, if you're experiencing stressful life events which could increase your risk of becoming addicted, you may wish to avoid using marijuana altogether—at least for now—since the risks could be far greater than any relief or pleasure you might reasonably hope to experience from using the drug.

17

Cannabis – Psychosis – Schizophrenia

Can cannabis lead to psychosis or schizophrenia?

> "I learned that courage was not the absence of fear, but the triumph over it. The brave man is not who that does not feel afraid but he who conquers that fear."

—Nelson Mandela

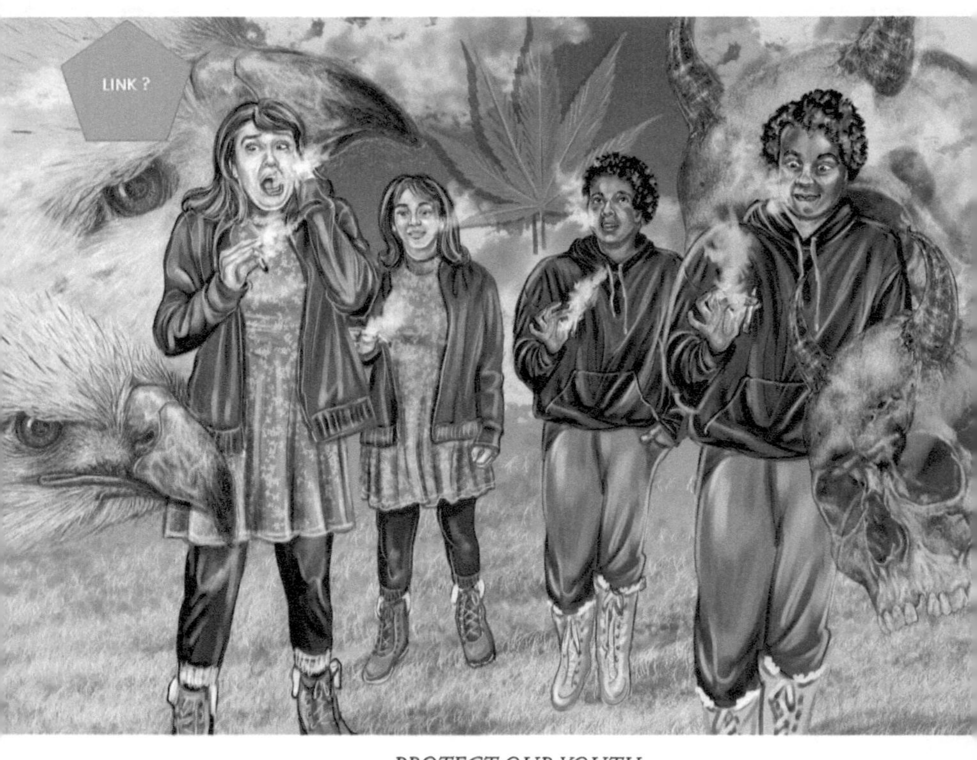

PROTECT OUR YOUTH
The 21 Unspoken Truths About Marijuana

> **Can I take cannabis if I am a teenager?**
>
> **Can I take cannabis if I am under 25 years old?**
>
> **The answer to these questions is: not without a potentially big risk!**

Can using cannabis lead to a psychotic episode or onset of schizophrenia?

Young lives can indeed sometimes be cut short by marijuana abuse, as this story illustrates: at the time of his death he was thirty years old, an aspiring song writer, and a great guy who is still missed by his friends to this day. From the first time he smoked pot, he experienced symptoms of psychosis as he repeatedly lost contact with reality, and believed himself to have super powers and was paranoid with feeling of persecution. These psychotic episodes could last between a few hours to a few weeks, but during his last time using marijuana, he took such a large amount of the drug that his judgement was completely distorted, and believing himself to be invincible and immortal, the man jumped from a dangerous height. All of a sudden this fine young man was gone.

In answer to the question: Yes, cannabis is associated with symptoms of psychosis which—for some people—can last a few hours, days, or weeks, and has been shown to trigger the early onset of certain types of psychotic disorders such as schizophrenia, whose symptoms might never go away.

How does Cannabis sometimes lead to symptoms of psychosis?

Among the approximately five-hundred chemicals found in marijuana, tetrahydrocannabinol (THC) is the chemical known to be most responsible in triggering symptoms of psychosis. Cannabis -or specifically THC- alters the functioning of parts of the brain known to be more involved in psychosis, for example it affects communication between parts of the brain called the prefrontal cortex and striatum. THC may also alter the balance of dopamine and other neurotransmitters within different parts of the brain, all of which creates a fiasco in your brain and changes the way your brain perceives reality and sensory information.

You may experience hallucinations while taking the drug (seeing things which are not there, or hearing sounds or voices which are inexistent). You may also find yourself having heightened attention or focusing on irrelevant details around you, resulting in your misinterpretation of other people's behavior (for example, thinking that people are plotting against you, are following you, or are spying on your behavior). You might also develop delusional beliefs, such as thinking that stories on the radio or television are secretly talking about you, or that the police is following or recording your every move. You might also believe yourself to be someone you're not as you disconnect more and more from reality.

Stats Corner

- The risk of psychosis is about 3% in the general population

- The risk of psychosis increases up to 2 to 5 times higher for regular and heavy cannabis users. [25, 26, 27, 41 44]

- Teenagers and young adults are much more at risk of psychosis when they use cannabis than adults

-Teenagers and young adults are at increased risk of falling into cannabis addiction than adults, therefore at increased risk of using cannabis regularly and consequently at increased risk of psychosis.

Again, if you're a teenager or a young adult under 25 years old, have other risk factors for developing an addiction, or have a family history of psychosis or other mental disorders, if you had a psychotic episode in the past, if you are a highly anxious or suspicious person, if you have a paranoid personality or have other mental illness, it's recommended that you exercise extreme caution and I highly recommend that you avoid trying marijuana since you are at a heightened risk of developing psychotic symptoms if you try cannabis.

Why unnecessarily risk deteriorating your mental health in a way which you might never be able to reverse?

Stats corner

- **Cannabis increases the risks of triggering a first episode of schizophrenia**

- **Cannabis may trigger symptoms of schizophrenia at an earlier age in life than would have otherwise been the case.**

- **50% of people who experience a toxic psychosis (psychosis resulting from consuming drugs) will develop a chronic psychotic disorder such as schizophrenia within the next ten years.**[27]

18

Cannabis - Lung Cancer

Could smoking cannabis cause lung cancer or other respiratory diseases?

"The only impossible journey is the one
you never begin."

—Anthony Robins

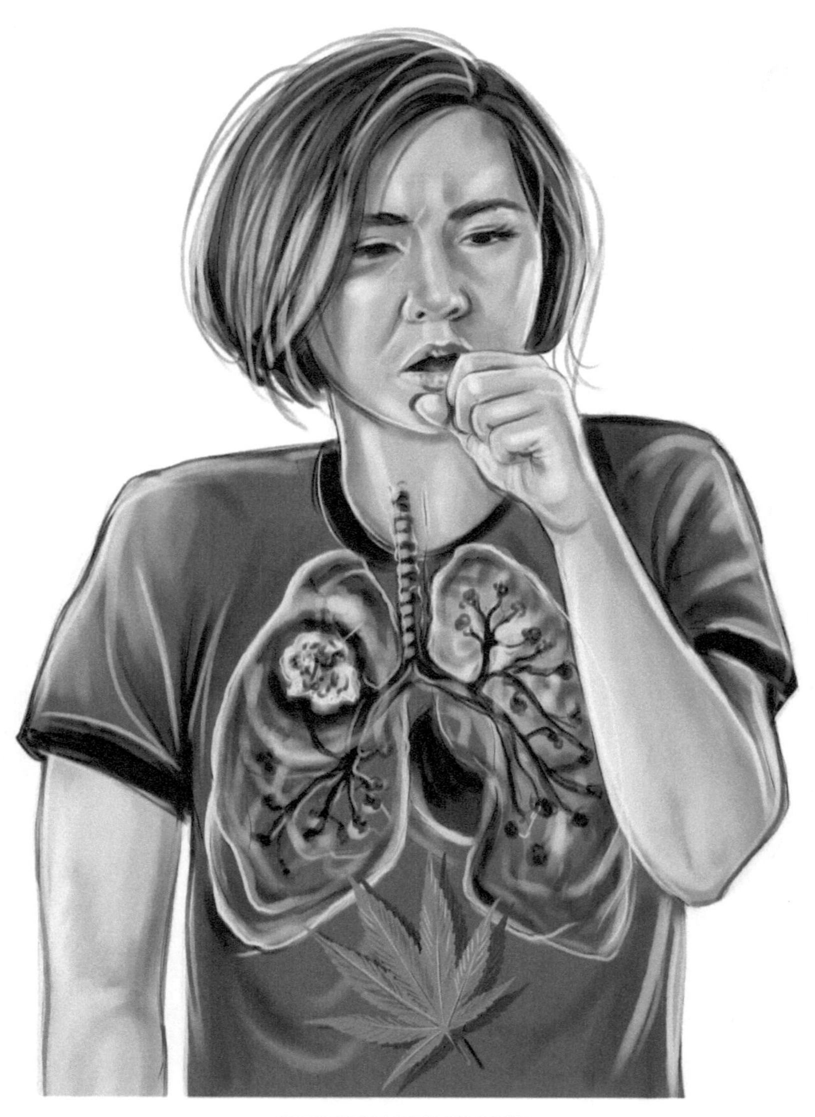

PROTECT OUR YOUTH
The 21 Unspoken Truths About Marijuana

Could smoking cannabis cause lung cancer or other respiratory diseases?

Let us picture a wonderful young sixteen-year-old girl suffering from severe asthma who chooses to smoke cannabis, and thereby ends up hospitalized in the emergency room, and potentially even risking death from an exacerbated asthma attack!

Frequent and heavy marijuana smokers often have respiratory problems such as shortness of breath, and increased sputum production in their lungs due to damage to their respiratory airways… similar to the symptoms seen in heavy tobacco smokers!

It's common knowledge that smoking tobacco is associated with many kinds of cancer especially lung cancer and other respiratory diseases. According to the American Thoracic Society[28] marijuana smoke contains many of the same harmful chemicals as tobacco smoke. And for people who already have respiratory conditions such as asthma, chronic bronchitis, and emphysema, smoking marijuana could worsen these conditions in much the same ways smoking cigarettes would.

Marijuana smoke contains over 450 chemicals and a lot of cancer causing chemicals similar to tobacco smoke.[28] So if tobacco smoke is widely known to increase the risk of lung cancer, and marijuana smoke has many similar cancer causing chemicals (carcinogens), it will be very fair to conclude that Marijuana smoke increases significantly the risk of lung cancer.

Smoke is smoke

*Cannabis smoke is very chemically similar to tobacco smoke

*They both contain very similar cancer causing chemicals (carcinogens)

*Cannabis smoke may contain 50% more carcinogens than tobacco smoke

*Smoking about 4 cannabis joints is equivalent to smoking a full package of tobacco cigarettes in terms of damages to your lungs and overall physical health

19

Hot Shower Marijuana Syndrome-Cannabinoid Hyperemesis Syndrome (CHS)

"We must free ourselves from the hope that the
sea will ever rest. We must learn to sail
in high winds."

-Aristotle Onassis

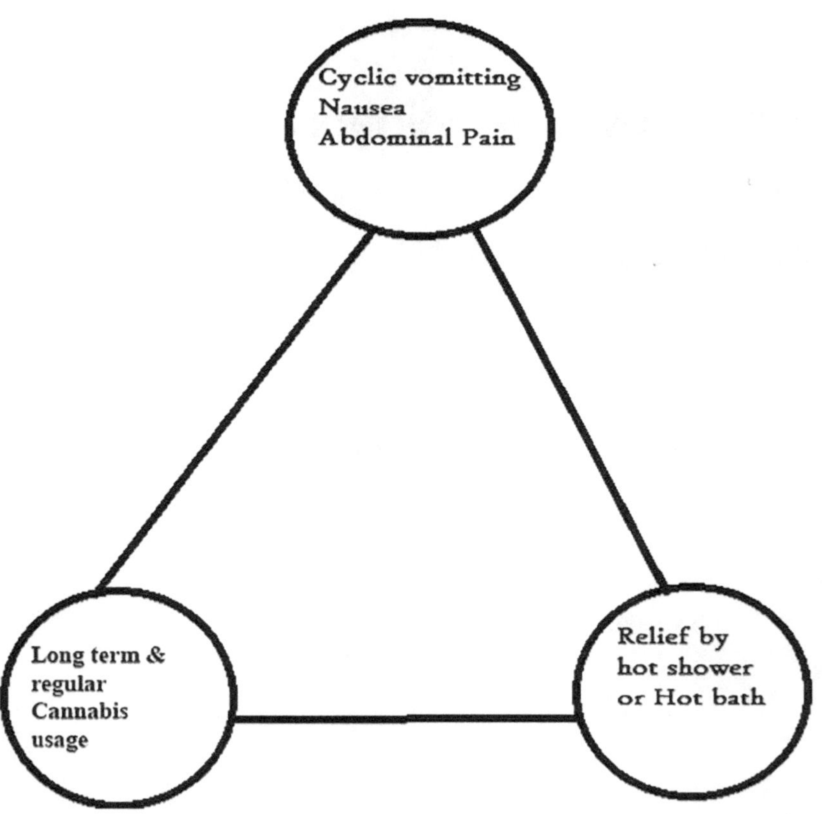

PROTECT OUR YOUTH
The 21 Unspoken Truths About Marijuana

HOT SHOWER MARIJUANA SYNDROME or CANNABINOID HYPEREMESIS SYNDROME

Let's say you or your friend, your kids or partner started to experience recurrent episodes of nausea and vomiting. You assume it's a gastrointestinal infection or food intoxication and it will pass, but it doesn't, it keeps coming back way too often and you finally decide to go see a doctor. They do all the necessary tests but they can't find anything and the doctors desperately tell you that it might be your anxiety causing those symptoms and they refer you to a psychiatrist who conclude that you need to be investigated more because your symptoms are not caused by anxiety.

In the process of trying to find solutions to ease your symptoms, you realize that a hot shower or bath relieves the symptoms of nausea, vomiting and vague abdominal pain, at least temporarily. And then you start taking showers many hours a day. Your family starts to get worried because you spend too much time in the shower, you start to get isolated and the electricity bill has increased exponentially due to frequent long hot showers and baths.

The situation becomes even more alarming when you start to get burns on your body due to too hot showers. You go to the ER to check with a doctor and you explain the whole situation and the doctor finally does the urine test to find out that cannabis is positive and asks you about your cannabis usage.

Cannabinoid Hyperemesis Syndrome

> **Almost 3 million Americans consulting in the emergency department might be suffering from cannabinoid hyperemesis syndrome.**[60]
>
> **In Colorado, the consultations for cyclic vomiting in the emergency department have doubled after legalization of recreational cannabis.**[58]
>
> **According to Canadian Institute of Health Information, the number of cannabis-related visits to emergency rooms has significantly increased in the last few years and most visits are related to palpitations and vomiting caused by cannabis.**

The case above illustrates well real cases seen in the ER and often mistaken for food poisoning or gastrointestinal infection. Cannabinoid Hyperemesis Syndrome that I also call *Hot Shower Marijuana Syndrome* is characterized by frequent and recurrent episodes of nausea, severe vomiting and vague abdominal pain in patients who have been using cannabis heavily and for a long time, for at least one or two years. These symptoms are not relieved by classics antiemetic (anti-nausea/vomiting) medications but they are mysteriously relieved by hot showers or baths; so patients suffering from this syndrome will usually take very hot showers or baths which can last many hours a day. It turns into an obsession and a compulsive behavior, and the person starts to feel bad if they can't easily have access to a shower or bath and this might result in isolation and the loss of employment; in some cases in the United States, it has led to bankruptcy due to frequent consultations, and elevated electricity and hot water bills.

The prevalence of this syndrome is not yet known, but a study suggests that almost 3 million Americans consulting in the emergency department might be suffering from cannabinoid hyperemesis syndrome.[60] According to Canadian Institute of Health Information, the number of cannabis-related visits to emergency rooms has significantly increased in the last few years and most visits are related to palpitations and vomiting caused by cannabis. Calls to poisoning control centers have significantly increased following legalization of cannabis in Canada. In Colorado, the consultations for cyclic vomiting in the emergency department have doubled after legalization of recreational cannabis.[58]

Cannabinoid Hyperemesis Syndrome (CHS) or Hot Shower Marijuana Syndrome

signs:

* **Cyclic nausea, vomiting (that can go up to 20 times per day), abdominal pain**
* **Symptoms not relieved by classic antiemetic medications**
* **No diarrhea is associated with the symptoms**
* **Symptoms temporarily relieved by hot bath or hot shower,**
* **so patients develop an obsession and compulsive behavior of taking hot baths/showers many hours per day**
* **symptoms associated with chronic and heavy cannabis usage**
* **symptoms stop when one stops cannabis usage.**

The pathophysiological mechanisms of this syndrome are not well known but a few hypotheses remain plausible. We know that cannabis binds to cannabinoid receptors in your brain, and these receptors are also present in your digestive system or gastrointestinal nervous system. One hypothesis is that the accumulation of cannabis in your system might result in vasodilatation of blood vessels in the gastrointestinal system which will interfere with a proper functioning of the gastrointestinal system and then increase nausea and vomiting. Another hypothesis is that cannabis acts directly on the part of your brain that controls vomiting, the vomiting center or *area postrema* located in your brainstem. The accumulation of cannabis and overstimulation of cannabinoid receptors in this vomiting center of the brain could increase nausea and vomiting.

We still don't have any explanation to why hot showers and hot baths relieve the symptoms, but a plausible theory is that a hot shower or hot bath increases vasodilatation (dilatation of blood vessels) of the skin, which helps in redistribution of the blood diverting it from the gastrointestinal system and thus reducing congestion there.

What is the treatment of Cannabinoid Hyperemesis Syndrome?

While hot showers or baths might temporarily reduce the symptoms, this is not a treatment at all, but a compulsive behavior developed to reduce the discomfort caused by abdominal pain, nausea and vomiting. The patient will be treated by hydration and correction of electrolytes imbalances caused by vomiting. The classic anti-emetic medications do not work for this syndrome.

Finally, the only way to stop the Cannabinoid Hyperemesis Syndrome or the Hot shower Marijuana Syndrome is by stopping cannabis altogether. When people stops cannabis, the symptoms disappear.

The only definitive treatment option is: stopping cannabis
Hydration will be used for dehydrated patients due to severe vomiting
Classic antiemetic medications are not efficient for this syndrome

---

20

Can Cannabis Be Lethal?

"The greatest glory in living lies not in never falling, but in rising every time we fall."

—Nelson Mandela

Marijuana overdose, not deadly, But....

This is a tough question worth considering. While almost all medical experts agree that you can't die from a marijuana overdose, the argument can be made that marijuana can kill, at least through indirect causes.

Yes, high doses of marijuana might cause an increase in heart rate which might result in increased risk of heart attack for vulnerable patients, especially those with previous heart conditions; Cannabis might cause a drop in blood pressure which may increase the risk of fainting or passing out, but these increases are usually temporary in nature. As the body gets used to the effects of marijuana these physical effects tend to decrease. While high doses of marijuana can be fatal, they are rarely directly associated with cardiac arrests, heart attacks, or strokes. Marijuana overdose therefore cannot be considered directly lethal.

Marijuana – cannabis - smoke might:

- increase heart rate, which might result in increased risk of heart attack, especially for those with previous heart conditions [42]

- increase the risk of stroke especially for the most vulnerable people with previous medical conditions

- cause the drop of blood pressure, which might result in increased risk of fainting or passing out [42]

- might cause damage to your blood vessels and consequently increase the risk of other associated medical conditions down the raod. [43]

Yet a doubt still remains; what do we tell the mother of the 30-year-old man who experienced marijuana induced psychotic episodes discussed in chapter 17? This man had been fit, strong, hard-working, and wanted to enjoy life to the fullest, but since he began consuming marijuana he has been regularly hospitalized numerous times with psychotic symptoms.

This man didn't take any other drugs at all. He was doing fine, had been working on a regular basis, was considered by his friends to be a funny person, but would continually decide to start taking marijuana again, despite all the consequences he had experienced.

In search of a bigger "buzz", he smoked a little bit more than he was used to one evening, and feeling invincible, he jumped from a great height, his perception and judgment affected, and believing himself to be invincible and immortal and able to survive the jump. This lovely young man died at the scene and now he is gone forever.

Now the question is what killed him? He didn't commit suicide, and had no intention to die; he just smoked cannabis because he wanted to feel great, to enjoy life, and he didn't take any other drugs or excessive alcohol. While the week before he had been feeling great—completely normal and well-functioning—now he is gone. So what really killed him, and what is the cause of his death? It is up to the reader to answer for themselves, but one can argue that Marijuana was responsible for his death.

Can I predict how I will react to cannabis?

You cannot predict with certainty how each individual will react to taking cannabis for the first time, and it can be difficult to predict how you may react even if you've used the drug in the past. You might react fine this time, yet react badly the next time. You cannot rule out the possibility that using marijuana might lead you down the road towards feeling depressed, might trigger a psychotic episode, or could lead to dependency issues and addiction. If you are at risk of mental health problems, you may even experience psychotic or suicidal thoughts the next time you try it!

> **You cannot know if your next experience will be like the last! You can never be one-hundred percent certain how you will react, any time you take cannabis or any other drug.**

You cannot know if the next experience will be like the last. You cannot say: "I've been smoking for many years and have never had a bad experience, and never experienced a psychotic episode, so I will keep smoking and will never have a bad experience in the future". If during any particular session you increase the consumed dosage, the concentration of the product you are using happens to be stronger, or you happen to increase your frequency of use for a certain time period, you cannot predict how your brain and body might react to these changes in the amount of cannabis you put in your body....

> **Every time you put addictive drugs into your body, you are putting a certain stress on your brain, and at some point you might experience a reaction you've never experienced before. These reactions might include psychosis, anxiety, depression, suicidal thoughts or dangerously deadly behaviors.**

21

Cannabis – Car Accidents & Workplace Safety

Does cannabis increase the risk of car accidents?

"Accidents, and particularly street and highway accidents, do not happen - they are caused."

—Ernest Greenwood

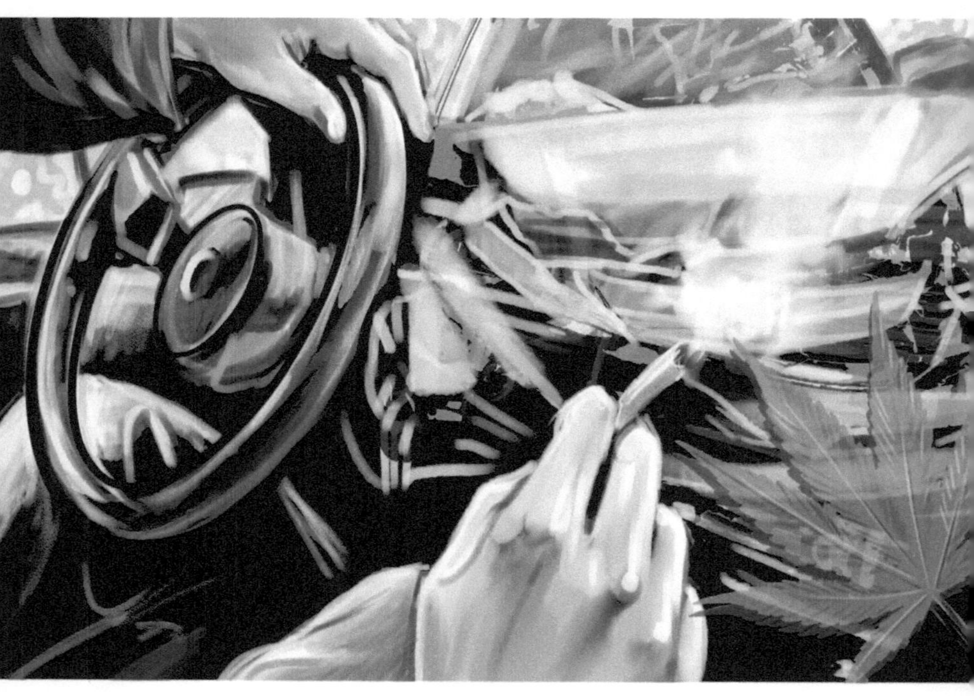

PROTECT OUR YOUTH
The 21 Unspoken Truths About Marijuana

Stats Corner

In 2016, there were 37,461 deaths from car accidents on U.S. public roads.

In 2015, there were 1,858 Canadian deaths from car accidents.

In 2011, there were more than 30000 deaths on European Unio roads.

A study has found a 3% increase in car accidents within U.S. states that have legalized recreational marijuana [29]

Different studies found that drivers under marijuana influence were at least 2 times more likely to be responsible for accidents than sober drivers (drivers without alcohol, cannabis or any other drugs) [30]

Pulling out from our driveway to drive to work, to a restaurant, to visit friends, family, or someone in the hospital, our main goal is to reach our destination and to get there securely. We take all the necessary precautions to drive safely and avoid getting into an accident.

But we have no control over other drivers' actions and we are totally powerless over the way they drive! We can only hope that they will drive as safely as we do. We hope the other driver is not sleepy, is not under the influence of drugs or alcohol or intoxicated in any other way. The only control we have is to report any deviant driving to the police. And this we can do—and should do—regularly!

> **- Cannabis affects your brain and reduces attention, concentration, motor coordination, and balance.**
>
> **- These factors reduce the ability to drive safely and to react quickly to spontaneous situations which arise while driving.**[32, 33]
>
> **- Therefore, cannabis significantly increases the risk of car accidents on the road not only for those who use it but for all of us on the road!**[34]

Road safety is a very distressing concern for most people. As discussed in previous chapters, cannabis use affects numerous parts of the brain such as the cerebellum (involved in balance and motor control), the basal ganglia (involved in motor control and coordination), and the prefrontal cortex (involved in focusing, paying attention, behavioral inhibition, and other crucial functions such as decision making and intuitive thinking).

In simple terms, cannabis reduces attention, concentration, motor coordination, balance, and affects reaction time. All these factors contribute in the driver's reduced ability to drive safely and to react quickly in case of abrupt or emergency circumstances on the road.

So cannabis will alter your ability to drive — as alcohol and other drugs also are known to do—and should be completely avoided if you plan to drive.

*** Driving 'high' is as dangerous as driving 'drunk'**

*** Different studies found that drivers under marijuana influence were 2 to 7 times more likely to be responsible for accidents than sober drivers(drivers without alcohol, cannabis or any other drugs)[30]**

*** When cannabis is combined with alcohol, the risk of car crash is even higher, 15 times higher compared to sober drivers.**

*** I strongly advice to avoid driving for a minimum of 8 hours after your last cannabis usage.**

*** And for those using edible cannabis, avoid driving for a minimum of 12 hours after you've eaten or drank cannabis products because edible cannabis lasts much longer in your system.**

Cannabis and workplace safety

In terms of workplace safety, the risk of an accident at work is increased for people with substance use disorder such as dependence or abuse of alcohol, cannabis and other drugs. According to a Canadian provincial agency on health and safety in the workplace in Quebec, people with an addiction problem are five times more likely to make a claim for occupational injury, they are involved in work-related accidents two to three times more often than others, they are absent three times more often than their colleagues and their performance is thirty percent lower than that of their colleagues.

People with a Substance Abuse or Dependence

*** Are 5 times more likely to make a claim for occupational injury than their colleagues**

*** Are involved in work-related accidents 2 to 3 times more often than others;**

*** Are absent 3 times more often than their colleagues**

*** Their performance is thirty percent lower than that of their colleagues.**

If you work in construction and you smoke cannabis or drink alcohol before or during work, you have a reduced attention, concentration, altered movement coordination and balance, and a limited ability to react quickly to sudden situations, all this can increase the risk of falling from heights or getting hurt or hurting your coworkers with tools.

If you are a traffic controller or an air traffic controller, you must stay away from alcohol, cannabis, or other drugs because your use can put the safety of many at risk. You are a construction engineer and you must make important decisions about the bridge or the building under construction, stay away from any substance that may cause erroneous decisions that may compromise the safety of the public or other employees.

You are a cook or manipulate sharp objects, you put yourself at a high risk of an accident at work if you consume alcohol, cannabis or other drugs before or during your shift. You are a car mechanic you need your maximum attention, your maximum concentration, your coordination of movements for your own safety and the safety of your clients. You are a nurse or doctor, you need all your faculties to make good decisions, your attention and concentration are required to avoid the risk of an accident for you but also for your patients. So very important to stay away from cannabis and alcohol and other drugs for at least 8 hours before your shift and a minimum of 12 hours if you used edible cannabis.

*** Stay away from cannabis and alcohol and other drugs for at least 8 hours before your shift.**

*** And for those using edible cannabis, avoid eating or drinking cannabis products for a minimum of 12 hours before your shift, because edible cannabis lasts much longer in your system.**

*** If you're intoxicated from a substance, you might consider to stay away from work for days of weeks or even suspend work until a medical evaluation depending on the level of your intoxication.**

22

Can Cannabis Lead to Suicide?

"It is during our darkest moments that we must
focus to see the light."

—Aristotle

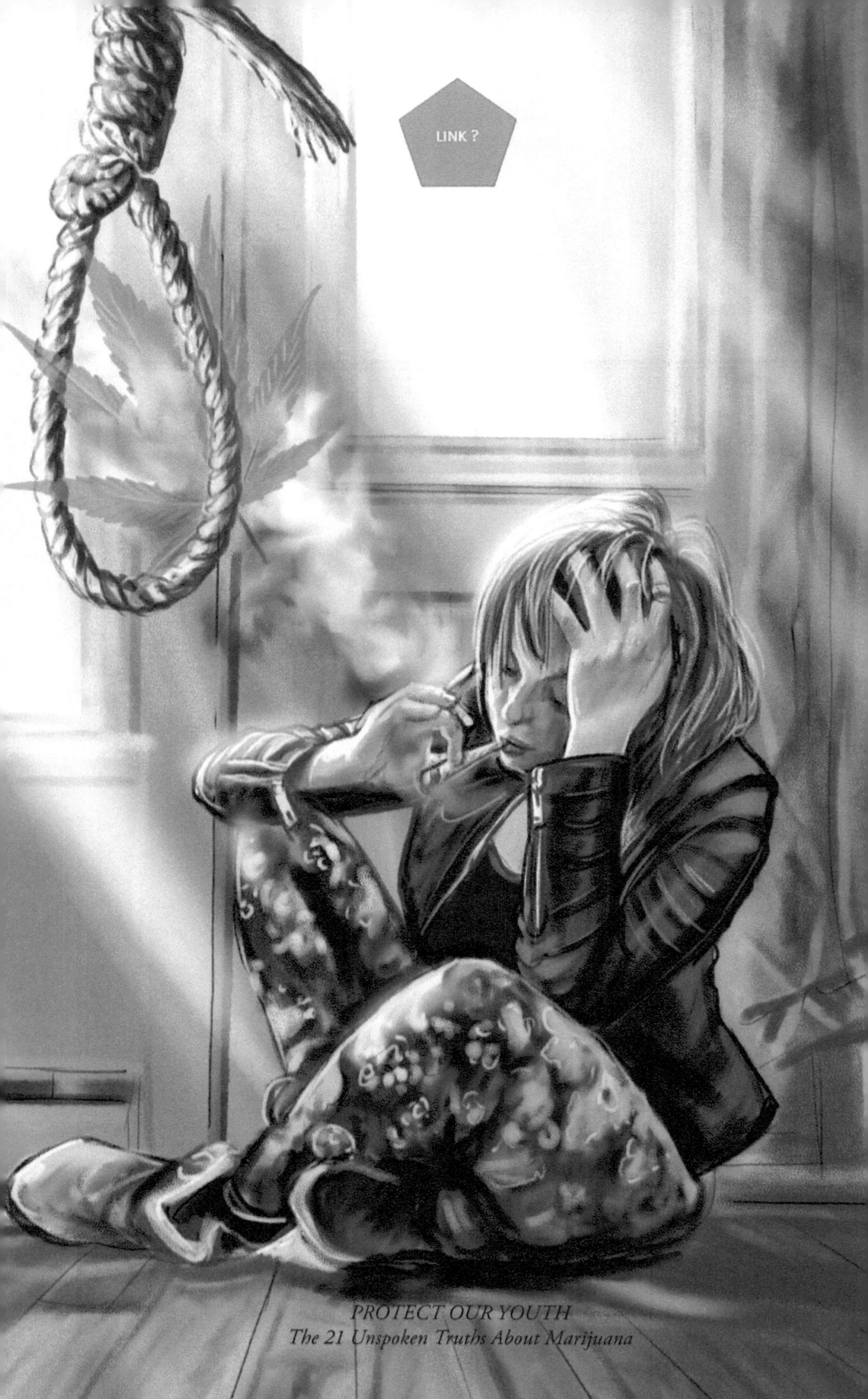

LINK ?
PROTECT OUR YOUTH
The 21 Unspoken Truths About Marijuana

> **Suicide often involves many accumulating stressful factors which put pressure on a person to the point that the problem seems irresolvable and the burden unbearable. The only way the person can envision escaping from the distress and suffering is through trying to end their life.**
> **Life still matters no matter what.**

Many factors such as physical illness, mental illness, financial stresses, bullying, divorce, academic or professional failure, social rejection, drug addiction, and sexual or physical abuse can all increase the risk of developing suicidal thoughts. There are studies which have suggested that regularly taking marijuana might also be significantly associated with increased risks of suicide (though all of these other risk factors may also play a role). But, why add yet another risk factor to your life?

> **Cannabis use among adolescents increases the risk of depression and suicidal behavior in adulthood.**[61]

This next paragraph will address the issue from another angle, but you can skip it if you're not interested in scientific theories linking cannabis use to increased risks of suicide. In down to earth terms, what happens to your brain when you take marijuana? Feelings of pleasure, euphoria, and the functioning of the brain's reward system are triggered when the brain's endocannabinoid system is activated; there are cannabinoid receptors in your brain and when you consume cannabis it binds to these receptors. However, some limited studies have produced results suggesting that people who died by suicide had a significant increase of cannabinoid receptors in some parts of the brain—especially within the prefrontal cortex—which could suggest that a hyperactive endocannabinoid system might be associated with increased risks of suicide![35, 36] However, it is important to emphasize that more research is needed in this area to be able to build up more solid conclusions.

Besides having direct physiological and behavioral impacts, we know that addictions to cannabis and other substances often point to signs of other emotional problems that we could be dealing with in potentially healthier ways. We might turn to pot to try to solve our search to define our personal identity, our desire to feel we belong somewhere, as an attempt to treat or medicate our symptoms of anxiety, as an attempt to suppress our painful feelings, to put forward a mask enabling us to seem happy and functional in social situations, or as an easy way to generate pleasurable feelings instead of utilizing more meaningful sources of pleasure. Suffering is always somehow present underneath the surface contributing to seeking out marijuana, and especially so when we find ourselves using it in abusive or addictive ways instead of facing our problems head-on.

> **Cannabis usage—especially when it slides into addiction— might be a mask we wear to cover the profound insecurity and the profound suffering and pain.**
>
> **But the more you indulge, the worse the pain, and the worse the pain, the more you indulge to soothe yourself. A cycle of personal negligence, lack of motivation, professional failure, and depression is triggered, leading you down the path towards hopelessness and potential suicidality. Still this tragic story can be avoided!!**

23

Proclaim Your Freedom, Reclaim Your Power!

"The best time to plant a tree was twenty years ago, the second best time is now."

— unknown

You feel like your freedom has been lost, and without realizing it, cannabis or other substances or habits have taken over your life, your family relationships, and your friendships. Your previous ambitions and personal dreams now seem unreachable. And you might be wondering how you can reclaim your power, how you can free yourself from addiction, and how you can become independent once more.

It might not be you, it might be someone you know, someone who is dear to you who is going through a period of loss of control over drug use or other addiction. You have a desire to help and you are wondering how to proceed.

> **You might be wondering how to free yourself from dependence and become independent once more. The point is to choose your own personal path towards your freedom, and to go for it!**

There is no straight path to conquering marijuana addiction (or any other addiction for that matter). Some people turn to self-help groups, others seek help from their doctors or psychotherapists, others participate in social, physical, or recreational clubs and activities, others join churches to try to rebuild their faith after having tried every other option. The point is to choose your own personal path to reclaim your freedom, and to go for it!

Here are five simple, yet challenging suggestions; why not give them a try, knowing that you can't succeed unless you start with one step at a time!

1. YOUR PROMISE, YOUR WORDS, YOUR FREEDOM

> **Your mind is a garden, everything you plant will grow**
>
> **Never cease to seed beautiful words in the garden of your mind.**
>
> **Use your mouth for you and not against you.**

At the beginning of what will realistically be a long battle, proclaim your freedom! The journey is not going to be easy, the battlefield might be harsh and cruel, but it's crucial to stay committed to staying on the frontlines. Dare to shout your commitment to becoming free; free indeed, free at last! Don't be afraid to proclaim to yourself—and to those closest to you—that you are taking responsibility towards concrete actions which will eventually result in your liberty. You are choosing to be free. Proclaim it over and over and over again!

> **Don't be afraid to speak out, to sing, to shout, and to repeat how free you are in the process of becoming.**

Let it sink into your mind, let it penetrate your soul; you have to create your freedom in your thoughts, words, and actions. Proclaim it loud and clear!

Your thoughts and words help create reality more than you can imagine. The way you think and speak about your experience of the world helps generate conflicts and the resolutions to conflict, apprehension and anxieties, or your confidence in your successes to come. Your words can create joy or sadness, and can either help build or destroy relationships. And of course, the way you use self-talk can help build up—or destroy— the vision and reality of who you feel yourself to be, and who you are to become in the world.

> **Choose to use your mouth to build yourself up, not to tear yourself down!**
>
> **Stop planting negative weeds, start planting flowers**
>
> **Stop planting despair, start seeding hope!**
>
> **Stop planting the past, start seeding the future**
>
> **Stop planting regrets, start planting contentedness**

Proclaim your victory immediately; don't be too shy to say "I'm a winner", and to voice the intention that you are on the right track. Every victory starts in your mind, before materializing in real life. Repeat this mantra as often as you can! Be dramatic about declaring how free you're becoming! Your thoughts and words about yourself—good or bad—are infinitely more powerful than the words coming out of anyone else's mouth. Your self-talk can either give you momentum, or they can stop you in your tracks. So be conscious about the thoughts and words you are putting into the world, and be careful with them, since they can have a lasting impact on the direction your life will be taking next!

> **- The only way you can create a habit of speaking good things into your own life, a habit of positive self-talk, is by doing just that over and over and over again, even when you don't feel like it.**
>
> **- Remember every victory starts in your mind, before materializing in real life.**

2. GET HELP

Get all the help you can, whenever you can, wherever you possibly can. Seek out all the support resources you have access to wherever you can find them, and as often as you possibly can. Whether it's through an in- patient rehab, out-patient rehabilitation center, self-help support group (for example, through Alcoholics' or Narcotics' anonymous, AA or NA groups), or church, there are numerous places we can go to, do not feel alone, dare to ask for help, search until you find. Try asking your doctor about available treatment options, go see an individual or group therapist, speak with your teacher, your coach, your nurse, your pastor, your priest, your religious leader, your life coach, your gym coach, your friends, your family, and see what feels right for you! Remember, you can't find what works for you if you aren't actively seeking out solutions. Again Search until you find. There are different services in different regions, inform yourself at your doctor's office or with your local officials about specific therapies available in your area for teenagers, young adults or for the adult population.

You never know who will be able to steer you in the direction which will ultimately work best for you… whether it's a health professional, support group member, doctor, therapist, friend, pastor, priest, or family member that helps you make the right moves, at the right time, remain open to new ways of getting help, and don't ever give up!

Don't be intimidated by your past

Don't let shame about your past dictate your future

Don't be humiliated by failures you might have along the way

Just remain willing to get up every time you fall, despite the challenges, and forever committed to turning each and every failure into a learning opportunity for eventual success!

Don't be satisfied with the status quo; search actively for answers, keep on standing up when you fall, don't wallow in feelings of shame, self-doubt, or self-pity! Remain willing to continue the fight and to go on, despite any challenge you might be facing.

Just remember that each day that passes by without you making efforts towards change means you'll be one day deeper into the problem. But once you've resolved to get help, forget about the comments naysaying friends or relatives who have negative things to say; you are investing in your life, and investing in your future. You are planting the seeds of change in your garden, and no one can take that away from you if you don't let them!

3. U-TURN, REVERSE, DELETE!

If your life is heading in the wrong direction, it's very hard to imagine how you will ever reach your intended destination. Realistically, it may take a drastic U-turn, a change in the right direction to be able to get there. Do you know what might that change look like?

Do you need to consider putting distance between yourself and those friends who are constantly pulling you down? Don't be shy to shy away from that social group who made it so easy to make unhealthy decisions; don't hesitate to delete them from your social media contacts, don't worry about erasing their names and numbers from your phone, and getting rid of your drug dealer's information. Don't hesitate to delete, delete and delete. Don't let yourself have regrets; sometimes we need to make difficult choices to reclaim our freedom.

> **Surround yourself with eagles that will help you fly, Don't be shy to shy away from those who pull you down**

4. NEW DISCIPLINE, NEW ROUTINE!

Build yourself a new routine and stick to it. Start eating healthy meals, and be determined to prepare food on regular schedule. Go to bed at a decent hour, and get up early with the rising sun! Start engaging in physical activities four to five times a week, and progressively start integrating more leisure and social activities in which there taking drugs isn't the primary focus.

New habits
With consultation and the help of your healthcare professional:

Sleep well: around 8 hours per night, go to bed early, get up early, avoid screens for at least an hour before going to bed, avoid caffeine after 2pm, maximum: 2 to 3 coffees per day if you can't avoid it altogether.

Move: Exercise: 30 – 45 minutes, 4 to 5 times per week

Drink water: around 2 liters per day

Eat well: regular meal at the table, not in front of the screens

Thinking habits: entertain advantageous thoughts, think different, think better than before.

Leisure activity : develop at least one leisure activity: sport, art, social club,…

Let's be clear: this is not going to be easy, it's actually going to be very challenging, but remember you're on the battlefield and it's not time to quit! Look for inspirational books, quotes, and advice that can keep you developing new habits of discipline, and learn to lean on your new healthier routines to stay strong and maintain your will-power in the face of hardships!

5. ENJOY THE "NEW YOU"!

This step is all about learning to live and enjoy your life, now that you've achieved sobriety. Cannabis or other drugs produces intense and quick pleasure, so it is not going to be ease to enjoy regular drug-free leisure activities, it is going to be a learning process. Don't hesitate to learn to enjoy again, it's by walking that we learned to walk. Don't hesitate to share how far you've come in a positive and encouraging way, and to let others know how great it feels to be free again! Try not to spend time dwelling on past regrets; instead spend more time shaping your present, and creating your future. Your new routine will be instrumental in learning new ways to enjoy your new life; meet new friends, get to know new acquaintances, explore and experiment with new drug-free leisure activities, and how the whole new you experience them!

- It is not going to be easy to enjoy regular drug-free leisure activities, it is going to be a challenging learning process. Don't hesitate to learn to enjoy again,

- Remember, it's by walking and falling and walking again that we all learned to walk.

- Dare to shout your commitment to becoming free; free indeed, free at last.

24

The 21 unspoken truths about Marijuana

I suggest that you take a brief moment to explore whether you have seized all the 21 unspoken truths about marijuana discussed in this book.

Have you grasped the links between Marijuana-Cannabis and:		
Psychosis/ schizophrenia	Depression	Anxiety
Suicide	Sleep problems	Cognitive dysfunction & ↓ I.Q. points
Car accidents	Antimotivational syndrome	Medical uses
Endocannabinoid System	Hot Shower Marijuana Syndrome/ Cannabinoid Hyperemesis Syndrome	Professional and school failure
Lung cancer	Blood vessel damage and heart problems	Safety in the workplace
Addiction risk	teenager's brain & young adults	Gateway drug or front door drug
Cannabis & Sexuality	Edible versus inhaled or smoked cannabis	Pregnancy & breastfeeding

References

(1) Freeman, A. (2017, April 13). Canada announces plans to legalize marijuana by July 2018. *The Washington Post.* Retrieved from https://www.washingtonpost.com/news/worldviews/wp/2017/04/13/canada-announces-plans-to-legalize-marijuana-by-july-2018/

(2) Center for Behavioral Health Statistics and Quality. (2016). *2015 National Survey on Drug Use and Health: Detailed Tables.* Substance Abuse and Mental Health Services Administration, Rockville, MD. Retrieved from https://www.samhsa.gov/data/sites/default/files/NSDUH-DetTabs-2015/NSDUH-DetTabs-2015/NSDUH-DetTabs-2015.pdf

(3) Leggett, T. (2006). A review of the world cannabis situation. *Bull Narc, 58*(1-2), 1-155.

(4) United Nations Office on Drugs and Crime. (2014). *World drug report 2014.* Retrieved from https://www.unodc.org/documents/wdr2014/ World Drug Report 2014 web.pdf

(5) Statistics Canada. (2015). *Canadian Tobacco, Alcohol and Drugs Survey (CTADS) 2015 summary.* Retrieved from https://www.canada.ca/en/health-canada/services/canadian-tobacco-alcohol-drugs-survey/2015-summary.html

(6) ER Visits for Kids Rise Significantly After Pot Legalized in Colorado (2017, May 5th), *NBC News.* Retrieved from https://www.nbcnews.com/health/health-news/er-visits-kids-rise-significantly-after-pot-legalized-colorado-n754781

(7) Center for Behavioral Health Statistics and Quality. (2013) *Drug Abuse Warning Network, 2011: National Estimates of Drug-Related Emergency Department Visits.* Substance Abuse

and Mental Health Services Administration, Rockville, MD. Retrieved from https://w w w.samhsa.gov/data/sites/default/ files/ DAWN2k11ED/DAWN2k11ED/DAWN2k11ED.pdf

(8)   Steinmetz, K. (2017, April 20th). 420 Day: Why There Are So Many Different Names for Weed. *Time Magazine*. Retrieved from http://time. com/4747501/420-day-weed-marijuana-pot-slang/

(9)   George, T., & Vaccarino, F. (Eds.). (2015). *Substance abuse in Canada: The Effects of Cannabis Use during Adolescence*. Ottawa, ON: Canadian Centre on Substance Abuse. Retrieved from http://www.ccsa.ca/Resource%20Library/ CCSA-Effects-of-Cannabis-Use-during-Adolescence-Report-2015-en.pdf

(10) Anthony, J. C., Warner, L. A., & Kessler, R. C. (1994). Comparative epidemiology of dependence on tobacco, alcohol, controlled substances, and inhalants: Basic findings from the national comorbidity survey. *Experimental and Clinical Psychopharmacology, 2*(3), 244.

(11) Lopez-Quintero, C., de los Cobos, José Pérez, Hasin, D. S., Okuda, M., Wang, S., Grant, B. F., & Blanco, C. (2011). Probability and predictors of transition from first use to dependence on nicotine, alcohol, cannabis, and cocaine: Results of the national epidemiologic survey on alcohol and related conditions (NESARC). *Drug and Alcohol Dependence, 115*(1), 120-130.

(12) Anthony, J.C. (2006). The epidemiology of cannabis dependence. *Cannabis Dependence: Its Nature, Consequences and Treatment*. Cambridge, UK: Cambridge University Press. 58-105.

(13) Committee opinion no. 637: Marijuana use during pregnancy and lactation. (2015). *Obstetrics & Gynecolog y, 126*(1), 234-238. Retrieved from https://journa ls.lw w.com/greenjournal/ Fulltext/2015/07000/ Committee Opinion No 637 Marijuana Use During.48.aspx

(14) Metz, T. D., & Stickrath, E. H. (2015). Marijuana use in pregnancy and lactation: A review of the evidence. *American Journal of Obstetrics and Gynecology, 213*(6), 761-778.

(15) Goldschmidt, L., Richardson, G. A., Willford, J. A., Severtson, S. G., & Day, N. L. (2012). School achievement in 14-year-old youths prenatally exposed to marijuana. *Neurotoxicology and Teratology, 34*(1), 161-167.

(16) Goldschmidt, L., Richardson, G. A., Willford, J., & Day, N. L. (2008). Prenatal marijuana exposure and intelligence test performance at age 6. *Journal of the American Academy of Child & Adolescent Psychiatry, 47*(3), 254-263.

(17) Volkow, N. D., Wang, G., Fowler, J. S., & Tomasi, D. (2012). Addiction circuitry in the human brain. *Annual Review of Pharmacology and Toxicology, 52*, 321-336.

(18) Merline, A., Jager, J., & Schulenberg, J. E. (2008). Adolescent risk factors for adult alcohol use and abuse: Stability and change of predictive value across early and middle adulthood. *Addiction, 103*(s1), 84-99.

(19 Zimmermann, P., Wittchen, H., Waszak, F., Nocon, A., Höfler, M., & Lieb, R. (2005). Pathways into ecstasy use: The role of prior cannabis use and ecstasy availability. *Drug and Alcohol Dependence, 79*(3), 331-341.

(20) NIDA. (2018). Marijuana. Retrieved from https://www.drugabuse.gov/drugs- abuse/marijuana on January 19, 2018

(21) Weinberger, A. H., Platt, J., & Goodwin, R. D. (2016). Is cannabis use associated with an increased risk of onset and persistence of alcohol use disorders? A three- year prospective study among adults in the united states. *Drug and Alcohol Dependence, 161*, 363-367.

(22) Meier, M. H., Caspi, A., Ambler, A., Harrington, H., Houts, R., Keefe, R. S., . . .Moffitt, T. E. (2012). Persistent cannabis users show neuropsychological decline from childhood to midlife. *Proceedings of the National Academy of Sciences of the United States of America, 109*(40), E2657-64. doi:10.1073/pnas.1206820109 [doi].

(23) Center for Behavioral Health Statistics and Quality. (2013) *Drug Abuse Warning Network, 2011: National Estimates of Drug-Related Emergency Department Visits.* Substance Abuse

and Mental Health Services Administration, Rockville, MD. Retrieved from https://w w w.samhsa.gov/data/sites/default/ files/ DAWN2k11ED/DAWN2k11ED/DAWN2k11ED.pdf

(24) Degenhardt, L., Chiu, W., Sampson, N., Kessler, R. C., Anthony, J. C., Angermeyer, M., . . . Huang, Y. (2008). Toward a global view of alcohol, tobacco, cannabis, and cocaine use: Findings from the WHO world mental health surveys. *PLoS Medicine, 5*(7), e141.

(25) Moore, T. H., Zammit, S., Lingford-Hughes, A., Barnes, T. R., Jones, P. B., Burke, M., & Lewis, G. (2007). Cannabis use and risk of psychotic or affective mental health outcomes: A systematic review. *The Lancet, 370*(9584), 319-328.

(26) Grant, C. N., & Bélanger, R. E. (2017). Cannabis and Canada's children and youth. *Paediatrics & Child Health, 22*(2), 98-102.

(27) Arendt, M., Rosenberg, R., Foldager, L., Perto, G., & Munk-Jorgensen, P. (2005). Cannabis-induced psychosis and subsequent schizophrenia-spectrum disorders: Follow-up study of 535 incident cases. *The British Journal of Psychiatry: The Journal of Mental Science, 187*, 510-515. doi:187/6/510 [pii]

(28) American Thoracic Society. (2017). *Smoking marijuana and the lungs*. Retrieved from https://www.thoracic.org/patients/ patient-resources/resources/marijuana.pdf

(29) Leefeldt, E. (2017, June 22). Legal pot and car crashes: Yes, there's a link. *CBS News*. Retrieved from https://w w w.cbsnews. com/news/ legal-pot-and-car-crashes-yes-theres-a-link/

(30) Elvik, R. (2013). Risk of road accident associated with the use of drugs: A systematic review and meta-analysis of evidence from epidemiological studies. *Accident Analysis & Prevention, 60*, 254-267.

(31) Center for Behavioral Health Statistics and Quality. (2013) *Drug Abuse Warning Network, 2011: National Estimates of Drug-Related Emergency Department Visits*. Substance Abuse and Mental Health Services Administration, Rockville, MD. Retrieved from https://w w w.samhsa.gov/data/sites/default/ files/ DAWN2k11ED/DAWN2k11ED/DAWN2k11ED.pdf

(32) Lenné, M. G., Dietze, P. M., Triggs, T. J., Walmsley, S., Murphy, B., & Redman, J. R. (2010). The effects of cannabis and alcohol on simulated arterial driving: Influences of driving experience and task demand. *Accident Analysis & Prevention, 42*(3), 859-866.

(33) Hartman, R. L., & Huestis, M. A. (2013). Cannabis effects on driving skills.*Clinical Chemistry, 59*(3), 478-492. doi:10.1373/clinchem.2012.194381 [doi]

(34) Asbridge, M., Poulin, C., & Donato, A. (2005). Motor vehicle collision risk and driving under the influence of cannabis: Evidence from adolescents in atlantic canada. *Accident Analysis & Prevention, 37*(6), 1025-1034. Retrieved from http:// www.bmj.com/content/bmj/344/bmj.e536.full.pdf

(35) Dwivedi, Y. (2012). *The Neurobiological Basis of Suicide*. Boca Raton (FL): CRC Press/Taylor & Francis. Retrieved from https://www.ncbi.nlm.nih.gov/books/ NBK107200/

(36) Serra, G., & Fratta, W. (2007). A possible role for the endocannabinoid system in the neurobiology of depression. *Clinical Practice and Epidemiology in Mental Health, 3*(1), 25.

(37) Asbridge, M., Poulin, C., & Donato, A. (2005). Motor vehicle collision risk and driving under the influence of cannabis: Evidence from adolescents in atlantic canada. *Accident Analysis & Prevention, 37*(6), 1025-1034.

(38) Carliner, H., Mauro, P. M., Brown, Q. L., Shmulewitz, D., Rahim-Juwel, R., Sarvet, A. L., . . . Hasin, D. S. (2017). The widening gender gap in marijuana use prevalence in the US during a period of economic change, 2002–2014. *Drug and Alcohol Dependence, 170*, 51-58.

(39) Rubino, T., Zamberletti, E., & Parolaro, D. (2012). Adolescent exposure to cannabis as a risk factor for psychiatric disorders. *Journal of Psychopharmacology, 26*(1), 177-188.

(40) Rey, J. M., Sawyer, M. G., Raphael, B., Patton, G. C., & Lynskey, M. (2002).Mental health of teenagers who use cannabis. results of an australian survey. *The British Journal of Psychiatry : The Journal of Mental Science, 180*, 216-221.

(41) Association des Médecins Psychiatres du Québec (AMPQ). *Legalization of Cannabis: Let's protect Future Generations.* position paper (2017, June 3). Retrieved from http://ampq.org/wp-content/uploads/2017/06/enonce-de- positionanglais1.pdf

(42) Thomas et al. (2014). Adverse cardiovascular, cerebrovascular, and peripheral vascular effects of marijuana inhalation: what cardiologists need to know. American Journal of Cardiology 113(1): 187–90. http://www.ajconline.org/ article/ S0002-9149(13)01976-0/fulltext

(43) Wang et al. (2016). One minute of marijuana secondhand smoke exposure substantially impairs vascular endothelial function. Journal of the American Heart Association. 5(8). https://w w w.ncbi.nlm.nih.gov/pmc/articles/ PMC5015303/

(44) Bourque J, Afzali MH, Conrod PJ. Association of Cannabis Use With Adolescent Psychotic Symptoms. *JAMA Psychiatry.* 2018;75(8):864–866. doi:10.1001/ jamapsychiatry.2018.1330

(45) Gregory B. Bovasso. (2001). Cannabis Abuse as a Risk Factor for Depressive Symptoms. *American Journal of Psychiatry.* 158(12), 2033-2037. doi:10.1176/ appi.ajp.158.12.2033

(46) Patton, G. C., Coffey, C., Carlin, J. B., Degenhardt, L., Lynskey, M., & Hall, W. (2002). Cannabis use and mental health in young people: cohort study. *BMJ.*2002; 325:1195. doi:10.1136/bmj.325.7374.1195

(47) Wittchen, H.-U., Fröhlich, C., Behrendt, S., Günther, A., Rehm, J., Zimmermann, P., . . . Perkonigg, A. (2007). Cannabis use and cannabis use disorders and their relationship to mental disorders: A 10-year prospective- longitudinal community study in adolescents. *Drug & Alcohol Dependence.*2006; 88, S60-S70. doi:10.1016/j.drugalcdep.2006.12.013

(48) Coffey, C., & Patton, G. C. (2016). Cannabis Use in Adolescence and Young Adulthood: A Review of Findings from the Victorian Adolescent Health Cohort Study. *Can J Psychiatry.* 2016 Jun; 61(6): 318-27. doi:10.1177/0706743716645289

(49) Hayatbakhsh, M. R., Najman, J. M., Jamrozik, K., Mamun, A. A., Alati, R., & Bor, W. (2007). Cannabis and Anxiety and

Depression in Young Adults: A Large Prospective Study. *Journal of the American Academy of Child & Adolescent Psychiatry.* 2007; 46(3), 408-417. doi:10.1097/chi.0b013e31802dc54d

(50) Degenhardt, L., Hall, W., & Lynskey, M. (2003). Exploring the association between cannabis use and depression.*Addiction.* 2003; 98(11), 1493-1504. doi:10.1046/j.1360-0443.2003.00437.x

(51) Fergusson, D. M., Horwood, L. J., & Swain-Campbell, N. (2002). Cannabis use and psychosocial adjustment in adolescence and young adulthood. *Addiction.* 2002 Sep; 97(9):1123-35. doi:10.1046/j.1360-0443.2002.00103.x

(52) Windle, M., & Wiesner, M. (2004). Trajectories of marijuana use from adolescence to young adulthood: Predictors and outcomes. *Development and Psychopathology.* 2004; 16(4), 1007-1027. doi:10.1017/S0954579404040118

(53) Crippa, J. A., Zuardi, A. W., Martín-Santos, R., Bhattacharyya, S., Atakan, Z., McGuire, P., & Fusar-Poli, P. (2009). Cannabis and anxiety: a critical review of the evidence. *Human Psychopharmacology.* 2009 Oct; 24(7), 515-523. doi:10.1002/hup.1048

(54) *Gray KM, Watson NL, Carpenter WJ, et al. N-acetylcysteine (NAC) in young marijuana users: an open-label pilot study. Am J Addict. 2010;19:187-189.*

(55) *Sheryl A. Ryan,MD,FAAP, Seth D. Ammerman,MD, FAAP, FSAHM, DABAM,Mary E. O'Connor,MD, MPH,FAAP (2018). Marijuana use during pregnancy and breastfeeding, implication for Neonatal and childhood Outcomes. American Academy of Pediatrics, Volume 142. Number 3, Septemember 2018: e20181889*

(56) *Centers for Disease Control and Prevention (CDC): Today's Heroin Epidemic. Retrieved from: https://www.cdc.gov/vitalsigns/heroin/index.html*

(57) Patterson DA, Smith E, Monahan M, et al. Cannabinoid hyperemesis and compulsive bathing: a case series and paradoxical pathophysiological explanation. J Am Board Fam Med. 2010;23(6):790–793.

(58) Fleming JE, Lockwood S. Cannabinoid Hyperemesis Syndrome. *Fed Pract.* 2017 Oct;34(10):33-36. PubMed PMID: 30766236; PubMed Central PMCID: PMC6370410.

59) Kim, H. S., Anderson, J. D., Saghafi, O., Heard, K. J., & Monte, A. A. (2015). Cyclic vomiting presentations following marijuana liberalization in Colorado. *Academic emergency medicine: official journal of the Society for Academic Emergency Medicine, 22*(6), 694–699. doi:10.1111/acem.12655

(60) Habboushe J1, Rubin A1, Liu H1, Hoffman RS1 The Prevalence of Cannabinoid Hyperemesis Syndrome Among Regular Marijuana Smokers in an Urban Public Hospital. Basic Clin Pharmacol Toxicol. 2018 Jun;122(6):660-662. doi: 10.1111/bcpt.12962. Epub 2018 Feb 23.

(61) Gobbi G, Atkin T, Zytynski T, et al. Association of Cannabis Use in Adolescence and Risk of Depression, Anxiety, and Suicidality in Young Adulthood: A Systematic Review and Meta-analysis. JAMA Psychiatry. Published online February 13, 201976(4):426–434. doi:10.1001/jamapsychiatry.2018.4500

(62) Montreal hospital sees spike in children with cannabis intoxication (May 16, 2019) CTV News. CTV Montreal's Cindy Sherwin. https://www.ctvnews.ca/health/montreal-hospital-sees-spike-in-children-with-cannabis-intoxication-1.4426134

(63) Terrie E. Moffitt, Madeline H. Meier, Avshalom Caspi, and Richie Poulton. Reply to Rogeberg and Daly: No evidence that socioeconomic status or personality differences confound the association between cannabis use and IQ decline. PNAS March 12, 2013 110 (11) E980-E982; https://doi.org/10.1073/pnas.1300618110